The Book of
Menopause

THE BOOK OF

men

pa

THE EDITORS OF
OPRAH DAILY
INTRODUCTION BY
OPRAH WINFREY

Real Talk, Real Science, Real Strategies for Your Next Chapter

Conter

ts

THE BIG M

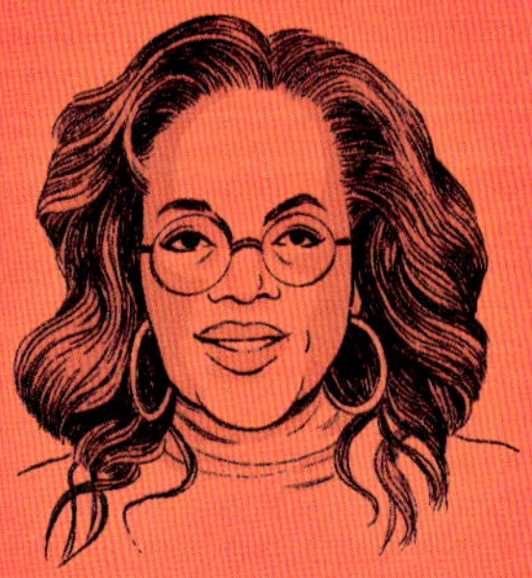

BY
OPRAH
WINFREY

For generation after generation, the word *menopause* was barely even whispered.

My mother's generation said not one thing about it. Even women who were just a little older than I am, no matter the symptoms, no matter the discomfort, they just endured it.

But there has been a radical shift in the past few years—you can feel it, can't you? Women are talking about menopause, and not just among themselves over coffee or school drop-off: They're giving TED Talks about the health consequences of this midlife shift. They're speaking out to Congress. Actresses who've traditionally spent their careers trying to look younger and sexier are now sharing their stories of inconvenient hot flashes, starting companies to create products to help, and advocating elected officials for more research funding. Friends are setting up text threads to share symptoms. Even men—men!?!?—are talking about menopause.

I can hardly believe it.

Now, I've been talking about The Change since I was 48 years old and first going through it myself. I've learned so much—but I'm still learning things that just completely blow my mind. For instance, menopause doesn't just cause a bunch of unpleasant symptoms. It affects *every single cell* of your body. Let that sink in!

That epiphany made me look back on my own experience through new eyes. I had heart palpitations that were so intense I couldn't sleep at night. For two years, I swear I hardly slept. I truly thought I was going to die. My journal was filled with "Wow, I made it through another night."

I went to five different doctors to find answers. Nobody knew what was going on. I was put on medication. I wore a heart monitor for weeks. And then one day, walking through the offices of *The Oprah Winfrey Show*, I picked up a copy of Dr. Christiane Northrup's book on women's health, and the pages fell open to the heading "Palpitations: Your Heart's Wake-Up Call." I took it as a sign.

Contained in that book was the answer I'd been going doctor to doctor trying to figure out. Heart palpitations and sleeplessness were indications that The Change was coming. But no one, including my trusted doctors, had warned me (did they even know?) and when my symptoms showed up, we looked for the most dire explanation—heart disease—instead of the most likely.

Until that point in my adult life, I don't recall one serious conversation with another woman about what to expect. Sure, I'd heard about hot flashes. But I wasn't prepared for heart palpitations. I wasn't prepared to have such difficulty concentrating. Reading, my favorite pastime, became a chore. Suddenly my attitude toward most things was "whatever." I wasn't vibrant. My whole world dulled down a couple of notches. When a friend mentioned that she'd felt the same dullness, and that her doctor had recommended an estrogen supplement, bingo. For me, too, that proved to be the answer. After I started hormone therapy, the world returned to technicolor. I could feel my countenance shifting. For the first time in years, I was sleeping the whole night through. At the time, I was ready to talk about it publicly, but back in 2001 when I tried to get any person of note to come on the show, there were exactly zero takers.

Still, I did multiple shows about my discovery for a few reasons. One, when I learn something, I want to share it so others can benefit, too. Also, there was so much shame at the time. People were embarrassed, confused, frustrated; some were even afraid to talk about menopause. They worried what people might think. They were concerned they'd be seen as old—too old to do their jobs, too old to date, too old to try something new. Sadly, there were so few research dollars dedicated to women's health, that like so many things, we had to fight hard to get answers. And then there were the Women's Health Initiative results in 2002, which because of the way the data was analyzed and reported caused a huge breast cancer scare and led to widespread discontinuation of hormone therapy—and a whole lot of misinformation—for generations to come.

Since then, we've learned much more about this crucial shift in our lives, so in 2023, I invited Gayle King, Maria Shriver, Drew Barrymore, Sharon Malone, MD,

Heather Hirsch, MD, and Oprah Daily Insiders to continue that conversation. Then I did another show on ABC, *The Menopause Revolution*, with Maria, Halle Berry, Naomi Watts, Mary Claire Haver, MD, and Rhonda Voskuhl, MD. And I continued the conversation on several episodes of my podcast.

Why? Because many women *still* feel shame or confusion or frustration about this phase of life. After each of these programs, I heard from so many of them. They continue to suffer through this natural part of life in silence with neither the guidance nor the resources to be prepared.

I don't want anyone to go through what I did, or to feel alone and confused about a transition that comes for all of us.

That's why I am so pleased to be sharing this book to help you navigate perimenopause and menopause. I am so grateful to all the experts who've shared their advice with Oprah Daily and O, *The Oprah Magazine*. Before we go any further, let me say this: I am not trying to replace the many wonderful menopause books out in the world. Truly—read them, underline them, gift them. We've got a whole reading list of them at the back of this book, because I want you to have *all* the tools.

What I *am* trying to do is give you a place to start. A place where you can get your bearings. Consider this book your lay-of-the-land guide. Your "here's what's real, here's what's changing, here's what you can do next" companion. My hope is that this book gives you a sense of what's going on in your body and your brain. What might happen in your relationships. What your treatment options are today—and what's potentially happening over the next few years. And yes, even what the men in your life are thinking.

My hope is that you'll find that menopause can be an opening, a shift toward yourself, where you get to step into a chapter defined not by what you lose, but by what you finally claim.

Start here. Take a breath. Then move through the chapters at your own pace. Let this continue the conversation we should've been having all along.

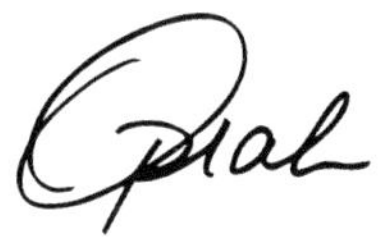

1

HORMO

NAL

BY **PILAR GUZMÁN**

HEALTH

Buckle up, things are about to get weird

A few years ago, at a cocktail party, I ran into an old friend who I hadn't seen since before the pandemic. It was 30 degrees out, though you would have never known it by her flushed cheeks and bare arms. She laughed, fanning herself mid–hot flash, and asked me if we could continue our conversation by an open window where she could cool down.

"They're like contractions," she joked about their mounting frequency. "Only there is no baby on the other side."

"You've started hormones, right?" I let slip and quickly regretted the unintended judgment in my tone.

"No, should I?" she asked. "My doctor said I didn't need them because my hormone levels were normal, though I feel like I've aged 10 years overnight."

"Yes," I said. It so happened that we were fresh off our live-audience taping in March of 2023 when Oprah convened some of the brightest minds in women's health to set the record straight on menopause and hormone replacement therapy (HRT). "It's not about treating the hot flashes, though hormones will help with that, too," I said, reiterating what I'd heard from Dr. Sharon Malone in that seminal conversation. "It's all the stuff you can't see—your heart, your brain, and your bones, all of which take a major hit when estrogen goes."

Since then I have had countless conversations just like this one with so many women—from those who go down all the medical rabbit holes and know how to advocate for themselves to the many more who don't. Regardless of socioeconomics, education, and degrees of entitlement, the story is almost always the same: A woman in her 40s or 50s goes in to see her gynecologist because she knows something is off. ("I just don't feel like myself" is the refrain from patients, wherever they are on their menopausal journey, according to gynecologist oncologist Elizabeth Poynor, MD.) She pushes past the shame, past all of the cultural conditioning that has taught her never to complain, and musters the courage to describe what's going on in her body: a seemingly random constellation of symptoms that can range from the most obvious (hot flashes, sleep disruption, and painful sex) to the more diffuse (frozen shoulder, tinnitus, and anxiety).

Invariably, she gets shut down with explanations like "Your hormone levels look fine" to "It's normal to feel this way" and maybe ends up with a prescription for an antidepressant. In this context, familiar narratives around "natural aging" and the idea that women have endured this for millennia without help take purchase, reinforcing a shame cycle that is the unique province of women.

This is happening despite the seeming explosion of menopause and perimenopause discussions. Yes, most Gen X and millennial women know that menopause happens on average at age 51, often right when we're finally figuring life out. We know it's preceded by perimenopause, a.k.a. the "menopause transition." We're aware that it involves hormonal fluctuations, beginning typically in our 40s (or as early as our 30s), and, unfortunately, that this phase tends to last on average four to eight years).

Although many of us know the basic facts—and certainly more information will be covered in this book—there's a lot we *don't* know about perimenopause and menopause. The reasons for that are both simple and complicated.

For starters, you might wonder why so many doctors are still so reluctant to prescribe hormones, despite all of the evidence pointing to their efficacy. One simple reason is that until relatively recently, there was a lack of training provided to doctors in medical school. It turns out, a whole lot of health care professionals are flying blind when faced with a sweating, sleepless, anxious 40-something patient. In 2003, a study found the topics of menopause and HRT were "almost nonexistent" in one medical school's curriculum. As recently as 2012, another study found that 80 percent of respondents reported limited training opportunities on menopause. So it's pretty easy to understand why otherwise terrific doctors might not be able to treat their menopausal patients confidently or share accurate, up-to-date information.

Another reason we don't understand the subtleties of the menopause transition is the flawed Women's Health Initiative (WHI) study Oprah mentioned. In 2002, it was stopped after it linked HRT to increased risks of heart disease, stroke, and breast cancer. Seemingly overnight women everywhere threw out their medication and decided to white-knuckle menopause instead.

The problem wasn't exactly that the WHI scientists were wrong about HRT, but that the results were misinterpreted and applied too broadly. The WHI mainly studied women who were, on average, in their early 60s, often more than 10 years past menopause. That's a very different group from the women who typically begin hormone therapy for symptom relief, who tend to be in their 40s or early 50s.

Looking closer at the data revealed that timing matters a lot. Starting estrogen many years after menopause can increase certain risks—like heart disease—but starting it earlier, closer to menopause, can actually be neutral or even protective. But the early headlines made it sound like hormone therapy was dangerous for *all* women, when really the risks were concentrated in women who started it much later in life. Women were spooked, doctors were spooked, and for the next 30 years, the standard of care around hormones became the smallest dosage for the shortest period of time possible.

More recent research has underscored the safety and efficacy of HRT (which now also goes by HT or MHT for menopause hormone therapy), including two game-changing studies released in 2025. The first, conducted by Mass General Brigham and published in JAMA *Internal Medicine*, looked back at 20 years' worth of data from 27,347 WHI participants who had hot flashes and night sweats. Researchers wanted to see if taking HRT at different ages could at all be linked to serious cardiovascular issues like heart attack and stroke. They found that women under age 60 who used HRT (which is what we'll call it in this book) did not have increased risk of cardiovascular issues. Another study of HRT started during perimenopause versus after menopause or not at all, found that women who began HRT within 10 years before menopause had no significantly higher risk of developing breast cancer, stroke and heart attack compared to the other two groups.

But that isn't the worst of it: Women were not routinely included in most major medical research until the 1990s. In fact, it wasn't until 1993 that the U.S. passed the NIH Revitalization Act, which finally required federally funded clinical studies to include women—and to actually analyze how sex differences might affect health outcomes. (They'd often been left out of trials due to a belief that fluctuating hormones made them too complex for study). This legislation essentially dragged medical research into the modern era, shifting women's health research from a narrow focus on reproduction to a more complete understanding of women's overall health.

Now, younger millennial women may think, "Well, the 1990s were forever ago, why do we still know so little?"

It hasn't actually been that long.

Think about it this way: Gen X women—your older colleagues, your hip aunties—got their periods not knowing about PMS. (That condition wasn't widely covered in the press until the late 1980s and early 1990s.) Gen X women had babies without knowing much, if anything, about postpartum depression. (Brooke Shields's memoir *Down Came the Rain* did start a larger conversation on the topic, but not until 2005, when many were in their 40s.) Gen Xers dealt with often painful and often confusing symptoms without ever hearing the terms polycystic ovary syndrome (PCOS), Premenstrual Dysphoric Disorder (PMDD), or Endometriosis.

We're not talking about grandmothers in scalloped-sided, black-and-white photos or mothers in Kodachrome home movies. We're talking about women of *The Breakfast Club* and *Thelma and Louise* era. Women who were told Title IX fixed everything, the first to be raised with the idea they could "have it all," and among the first to earn more bachelors degrees than men. They didn't even learn the word *perimenopause* until they were practically drowning in it.

If that weren't enough to grind your gears, consider that *if* the U.S. had launched a wide-ranging, long-term women's health study as part of that 1993 NIH act—something like Harvard's famous Framingham Heart Study that began in 1948 and followed thousands of men across multiple generations—we would now have a decades-deep better understanding of women's health.

Which sounds great and would be great, except when you realize that even if we had begun a study at that time with, say, college students, the first cohort of women would only just be entering menopause. (We do have the SWAN study, begun in the mid 1990s, but that's a long-term observational study of just 3,000 women designed to see what happens naturally, without testing any interventions.)

This makes it even more disappointing that the WHI study ended early. It was much bigger, with 161,000 women in randomized clinical trials, and focused on wider issues like cardiovascular disease, breast and colorectal cancer, stroke and blood clots, and more.

Can you imagine what else we could have learned and how much earlier we could have discovered it if the WHI study had continued?

Or can you imagine what we could have learned if we had been listening to women all along?

It always comes back to the same question for us here at Oprah Daily: Why aren't we as a culture more proactive when it comes to women's health at midlife? Why is it not standard medical practice to scan for the impacts of hormonal decline preemptively,

> "The real aha moment came from Elizabeth Poynor, MD, who said, 'Women's health is hormonal health.' She made us realize we'd been looking at women's health all wrong."

especially when we know that estrogen supplies are only moving in one direction? Instead we are operating on the defensive, waiting for a broken hip, a cardiac incident or "treatment resistant" depression before hormones get prescribed. As Dr. Jessica Shepherd says, "It's like waiting for your car to completely run out of oil before you change it."

We think it's time for a broader perspective. As Dr. Elizabeth Comen told Oprah, women's health has long been treated as "bikini medicine"—a narrow focus on the reproductive organs covered by a swimsuit. But that overlooks a number of conditions: autoimmune disorders (which disproportionately affect women), dementia (two-thirds of patients are women), and heart disease (our number one cause of death). In other words, the current model leaves out the majority of what actually matters.

The real *aha* moment around this faulty framing, though, came when we sat down with Elizabeth Poynor, MD for an interview and she said matter-of-factly, "Women's health *is* hormonal health." As a gynecologic oncologist and advanced pelvic surgeon who has spent her entire career managing some of the most complex women's health issues, her job has been to look at all of the systems of the body in relation to one another.

In this one simple statement she made us realize that we had been looking at women's health all wrong: Instead of viewing it as a set of separate chapters—menstruation, fertility, pregnancy, menopause—we realized we should be looking at the entire journey as interconnected. We need to move away from our current siloed thinking, which makes us believe we just have to get to the end of each phase so things can return to "normal."

Because there isn't one specific normal, is there? Our hormones are forever in flux—remember, that's the reason women were excluded from studies for so long. The upside, however, is that given half the population deals with these fluctuations, there are patterns—we are reliably in flux.

There seems to be greater acceptance of this variability in women during their reproductive years, but we still have lots of work to do to overcome assumptions that this same flux disappears with our periods. Remember, women spend 41 percent of their lives in a post-reproductive state. On the one hand, the so-called morbidity-mortality paradox tells us that while women live longer on average than men, they often experience higher rates of chronic disease and frailty in later years. On the other hand, we know that hormones help healthy cells all over the body stay healthy longer, and, statistically, hormone replacement increases not just lifespan but healthspan. You do the math.

Language matters, too. While we are thrilled that we are now talking openly about perimenopause and menopause, we're with Dr. Malone who says she doesn't like the term postmenopause. "To say you're postmenopausal means that you are over it. To say that you are over it means that you are no longer at risk for the things that we associate with menopause. But once you're menopausal, you're menopausal forever. Yes, some of the symptoms will get better, but the other changes that are going on in your body will continue from the moment you have your last period to the day you close your eyes."

Which is why we believe that looking at the whole spectrum of hormonal health will be more beneficial to women. Consider a 2020 meta-analysis of studies that found that women with PCOS have higher risks of major heart attack and stroke. Separate studies have discerned links between PMS or PMDD and earlier menopause with more severe vasomotor symptoms—hot flashes and night sweats. Other research finds women who had preeclampsia or gestational hypertension have a two to four times higher risk of heart attack and stroke later in life.

This and other research suggest that hormones tell a story about women's health that we've barely begun to listen to. By advocating for a hormonal-health approach, we're suggesting a model that finally matches women's lived experience—one where our physical, emotional, cognitive, and relational changes aren't treated as random symptoms but as connected responses to an underlying system.

This matters profoundly in midlife, when perimenopause and menopause bring some of the most dramatic hormonal shifts we'll ever face. Understanding those shifts doesn't just help us manage symptoms; it helps us understand ourselves.

In the chapters ahead, we'll look at what actually happens in your body and mind during this transition—and why it can feel like someone swapped out your operating system without warning. We'll talk about how these changes affect your energy, sleep, sex life, mood, and relationships and work. We'll go through the treatments, supports, and strategies that can genuinely help—and what it means when nothing seems to help at all. We'll explore how men think about this phase (yes, they have thoughts), what breakthroughs and new research are on the horizon, and why this moment in your life may actually be the beginning of a personal renaissance.

Because once we stop seeing perimenopause and menopause as an ending and start seeing them through the wider lens of hormonal health, the picture changes. What once seemed unpredictable starts to feel understandable—and manageable.

Pilar Guzmán is the editorial director of Oprah Daily.

what MENOPAU *does* BODY

USE

to your

2

Things that can happen when certain hormones have left the building

Menopause can feel as if the body—hormonally tipped off to the impending egg shortage—has launched into a panicky bank run, alarms blaring everywhere at once: hot flashes, joints on fire, parched vaginas, nights fractured by wake-ups and sweat. Brittle nails. Dry mouth. Migraines. But it can also arrive quietly. Just a few off-kilter periods with a side of forgetfulness that is the province of busy women at midlife. Or some completely different mix of symptoms altogether. (See page 52 for a loooong list of those).

The more clinicians listen, the longer that list seems to grow. Women describe itchy skin. A hip that suddenly feels locked. A body that no longer feels quite familiar. The reason doctors now connect so many of these complaints to the menopause transition is simple, says Sharon Malone, MD: "Because they weren't there before—and once you take estrogen, they go away."

That's not a coincidence. Estrogen receptors are everywhere: in the brain, the bones, the joints, the skin, the bladder, the gut. When estrogen levels begin to fluctuate and fall, the effects don't stay neatly contained in the reproductive system. They show up wherever those receptors live. Which is to say: almost everywhere.

Historically, many of these symptoms weren't linked to menopause because they can start years—sometimes a decade—before a final period. "A lot of times women wouldn't even think to complain," Malone says. "Because they're not thinking of menopause, and their doctor's not thinking of it, either." The result is a familiar pattern: skin issues sent to dermatology, anxiety to psychiatry, weight gain to endocrinology—each symptom siloed, each treated as its own separate problem.

What often gets missed is the larger picture. Malone urges women 35 and older—and the clinicians who care for them—to pause and ask a different question: *Could all of this be connected*? Instead of chasing symptoms one by one, a more comprehensive view can open the door to treatment plans that actually match what's happening in the body.

That might include a conversation with your ob-gyn and starting hormone therapy. It might also involve targeted exercise, dietary shifts, better sleep support, or stress management. Not every approach works for every woman, and not everyone can or wants to use hormone therapy. But for many, addressing the menopause transition holistically can make a meaningful difference across multiple symptoms at once.

This chapter focuses on the physical changes that accompany perimenopause and menopause—not just the ones that announce themselves loudly, but the quieter shifts that unfold over time. What follows is a guide to those changes—what's common, what's treatable, what tends to improve, and what deserves long-term attention. Think of it not as a checklist to panic over, but as a map: a way to understand what your body is doing now, what it may do next, and where intervention can help.

The Usual Suspects

Hot flashes, mood swings, sleep chaos, and other ways menopause announces itself.

HORMONES

When clinicians talk about the hormone shifts of midlife, they are usually talking about estrogen, progesterone, and, more recently, testosterone. Estrogen, the most influential, affects far more than reproduction. Its decline impacts temperature regulation, sleep, mood, bone density, cardiovascular health, vaginal and urinary tissues, skin, and brain function. Progesterone, which normally counterbalances estrogen during the menstrual cycle, also wanes, contributing to sleep disruption and cycle irregularity during perimenopause. Testosterone, produced by both the ovaries and adrenal glands, declines more gradually with age but plays a role in sexual desire, muscle mass, energy, and cognitive vitality; its importance in midlife health is now receiving increased clinical attention.

Because perimenopause typically starts four to eight years before menopause—and symptoms may persist for years into menopause, particularly without treatment—many women have become more interested in hormone therapy (commonly called HRT). When appropriately prescribed, it remains the most effective treatment for menopausal symptoms, eliminating approximately 90 to 95 percent of hot flashes and often improving sleep, mood, vaginal comfort, and overall quality of life. Evidence also suggests that initiating HRT during perimenopause or within 10 years after menopause may confer protection against osteoporosis, cardiovascular disease, and cognitive decline.

Hormone therapy is considered safe for most healthy women who are newly menopausal or within 10 years into menopause. Available in patches, pills, gels, sprays, creams, and vaginal rings, HRT uses substantially lower hormone doses than low-dose oral contraceptives. (Women with a uterus require progesterone alongside estrogen to reduce the risk of endometrial cancer.)

Generally HRT is avoided only for those with a history of hormone-dependent cancers, certain blood clots or strokes, liver disease, heart attack, or unexplained vaginal bleeding. But they don't need to suffer either; trained clinicians can point them to nonhormonal options to help address the symptoms of hormonal fluctuations. (You'll find more on hormone therapy and alternate treatments throughout these pages.)

WEIGHT GAIN

Weight gain is one of the most common—and most resented—features of the menopause transition. Not dramatic overnight changes, but a steady creep: roughly three pounds a year, adding up to about 20 pounds over time. For many women, it arrives despite no obvious change in eating or exercise, which is precisely what makes it feel unfair.

Part of the issue is where the weight goes. As estrogen declines, fat storage shifts toward the abdomen. Before menopause, abdominal fat typically accounts for about 5 to 8 percent of total body weight. After menopause, it can climb to 15 to 20 percent. This visceral fat sits deep around the organs and is closely linked to insulin resistance, heart disease, and metabolic dysfunction.

Insulin resistance helps explain why weight gain feels so stubborn: with lower estrogen, the body has a harder time turning food into energy, so more of it ends up stored as fat—particularly in the belly.

The reflexive response is to eat less. Smaller portions. Skipped meals. But chronic under-eating often backfires. Esther Blum, an integrative dietitian and menopause specialist, says many midlife women she sees are consuming 900 to 1,000 calories a day. That level of restriction can raise cortisol, destabilize blood sugar, and disrupt sleep, all of which spur weight gain. For most women in their 30s through 50s, baseline needs are closer to 1,600 to 2,200 calories a day, depending on activity.

What matters most is where those calories come from. Fiber-rich carbohydrates—beans, lentils, chickpeas, squash, rice, skin-on potatoes, and root vegetables—support adrenal health and blood sugar balance. Protein is equally critical, particularly during menopause, when muscle mass naturally declines. Maintaining lean muscle helps stabilize glucose, boost metabolism, and support energy levels.

This is where GLP-1 medications have entered the conversation. Drugs like semaglutide and tirzepatide have demonstrated meaningful weight loss and improvements in diabetes and cardiovascular risk markers. Emerging research suggests they may be particularly effective when paired with menopausal hormone therapy.

Hormone therapy doesn't cause weight loss on its own, says Stephanie Faubion, MD, director of Mayo Clinic's Center for Women's Health, but it may improve fat distribution and sleep, creating more favorable metabolic conditions. Women using both treatments also saw improvements in blood sugar, blood pressure, and cholesterol.

There are caveats. Larger studies are needed, and GLP-1 drugs don't reliably reverse menopausal fat redistribution. They're also associated with muscle loss. Which brings the conversation back to basics: resistance and weight training aren't optional. In midlife, they are foundational.

HOT FLASHES & NIGHT SWEATS

"I suffered many times with these wicked, wicked hot flashes," remembers Gayle King. "I was on a red carpet once, and a photographer asked, 'Gayle, you all right!?' They had to give me a towel!" Gayle is not alone: Up to 80 percent of women experience vasomotor symptoms (VMS)—hot flashes around their face, neck, chest, and upper back, plus night sweats. Typically starting in the late 40s, hot flashes and night sweats can last for several months or several years. According to a study in JAMA, the median length of the whole shebang is 7.4 years (roughly 3 before your last period and 4.5 after).

Some women, though, find hot flashes can last longer—a lot longer. "I've had patients experience VMS for one to two years [after menopause], and a handful continue to have hot flashes into their 80s, or even their 90s," says Tara K. Iyer, MD, MSCP, lead physician at Brigham and Women's Hospital's Menopause and Midlife Clinic and an instructor in medicine at Harvard Medical School.

How long they last can be affected by factors like race and ethnicity. For example, research presented at the 2022 North American Menopause Society's annual meeting found that Black women are more likely to experience severe hot flashes and night sweats for longer periods of time.

If you're going through an unavoidably stressful period in your life, due to divorce, grief, or financial issues, all of these psychological pressures worsen VMS, according to a research review.

Smokers also tend to suffer more episodes: In an analysis of 21,600 women around 50 years of age, smokers who were overweight were more likely to report hot flashes and night sweats. When those smokers lost weight, the incidence of VMS diminished, though not to the same levels of women who had never smoked. The good news: Women who quit smoking before they saw their 40th birthday experienced VMS symptoms to around the same extent as women who had never smoked.

So how to get relief? As always, speak with your doctor about treatment options. Hormone therapy has been shown to reduce symptoms by roughly 90 percent, but it isn't the only treatment option to consider. Mindfulness, breathwork and movement practices like meditation and yoga, and talking with a therapist can also be very helpful. "For women who can't safely have HRT, or don't wish to take hormone therapy, nonhormone medications may prove useful to reduce hot flashes and night sweats," says Iyer.

$340 MILLION

Between **1999 and 2011**, just one aspect of menopause, **vasomotor symptoms**—also known as VMS or hot flashes—**cost companies this much money annually.** Women who suffered from hot flashes made **1.5 million more health visits** than women who didn't experience them.

(SOURCE: A 2014 STUDY BY YALE SCHOOL OF MEDICINE RESEARCHERS)

In 2013, Brisdelle became the first FDA-approved, nonhormonal treatment for moderate to severe VMS. The active drug in Brisdelle is paroxetine, a selective serotonin reuptake inhibitor (SSRI), which, in higher doses, is used for depression (Paxil).

After that was approved, it was crickets for a decade. Then, in May 2023, the FDA approved another nonhormonal treatment called fezolinetant, marketed as Veozah. The first drug of its kind—a neurokinin 3 (NK3) receptor antagonist—it works by binding and blocking a receptor in the brain that regulates body temperature. Its high price tag, around $550 a month, may be due to its first-to-market status, but it won't be alone on the shelves for long. "Everybody's jumping into this hot flash treatment," says Stephanie Faubion, MD, director of Mayo Clinic's Center for Women's Health and medical director for the Menopause Society.

The latest nonhormonal newcomer is elinzanetant, which the FDA just approved to treat moderate-to-severe hot flashes and is available in the United States under the brand name Lynkuet. The drug blocks not one, but two brain receptors controlling body temperature; results from the clinical trials suggest that the drug might also improve sleep quality.

DRY, DULL, SAGGING SKIN

The four to 10 years leading up to your last period trigger a host of skin-related concerns. Studies show that estrogen plays a vital role in collagen production, elasticity, thickness, moisture levels, and healthy blood vessels. When it plummets during perimenopause, you start to see the opposite: dryness, dullness, lines and wrinkles, and sagging. It can feel like a roller coaster: Estrogen's downward trajectory—and its effect on your complexion—isn't gradual or gentle; it's a series of erratic spikes and crashes that leave you wondering if you aged 10 years overnight. "I can tell that a woman is in perimenopause when she comes to me and says, 'My skin just fell apart,'" says Doris Day, MD, a dermatologist in New York City.

When caring for her middle-aged patients, Miami dermatologist Leslie Baumann, MD, says, "I don't delineate between perimenopausal, menopausal, or postmenopausal—they all affect the skin similarly."

It's a good idea to have your hormone levels checked in your late 30s and early 40s, and discuss hormone replacement therapy options with your doctor. "HRT isn't right for everybody and won't solve all problems. But you will have a better chance of keeping menopause symptoms at bay and skin healthier while you're on it," Day says.

There's also plenty you can do topically to revitalize your skin. Here's our guide.

DRYNESS: This is a sign that your skin's outer protective barrier isn't up to snuff. As estrogen levels fall, the skin's epidermis thins, and your sebaceous glands become less active, reducing oil production. Not every sign of aging is caused by low estrogen—sun exposure, genetics, and time all play a part, but estrogen loss accelerates many of those changes. Switch to a mild or gentle cleanser that won't strip dry skin of its essential oils. Then shore up the skin's barrier with a moisturizer featuring ingredients such as ceramides, shea butter, fatty acids, squalane, glycerin, or hyaluronic acid, which add moisture and help keep it there. Same goes for your body: Use a creamy body wash and a body lotion with those same ingredients. There is a new crop of estrogen face and eye creams, as well. If you've ever used a vaginal estrogen cream, you've already seen what this hormone can do for skin. "Estrogen cream changes the anatomy of the vaginal tissue," says Somi Javaid, an ob-gyn in Ohio and founder of HerMD, a women's health care platform. "By replacing estrogen locally, you stimulate collagen, improve blood flow, and strengthen the skin's natural barrier."

DULLNESS: Menopause-induced dryness coupled with the lagging cell turnover that comes with age makes skin look lackluster. "This happens when dead skin cells heap up on the surface—under a microscope, it looks like hills and valleys," says Dr. Baumann. "That topography doesn't reflect the light so well." And light reflection is what gives skin a glow. Exfoliation is key to keeping skin looking luminous. Alpha hydroxy acids (AHAs) help slough off dead skin to reveal brighter skin. Glycolic acid, an AHA, is ideal because it's a humectant, which means it attracts moisture. Use a glycolic-containing serum every other day if your skin can tolerate it.

FINE LINES AND WRINKLES: The culprit here is the dwindling collagen supply. You start to lose about 1 percent of your collagen annually in your 30s, but that depletion escalates after menopause. "You lose 30 percent of your collagen in the first five years after menopause," says Dr. Day. "So it's important to keep building collagen while you still can. The fix? Two words: topical retinoids. "You don't need a prescription; these days, the OTC versions are effective and less drying," Dr. Day says. These vitamin A derivatives stimulate collagen production and rev up cell turnover, making skin noticeably smoother. Dr. Baumann also suggests applying a topical vitamin C serum and taking an oral vitamin C supplement (500 mg twice a day). The antioxidant vitamin is essential for collagen production. Be sure to follow with a moisturizer. Some formulas made for mature skin may help stimulate your body's estrogen receptors as well.

SAGGING: Just as collagen depletes with age, so does its partner elastin—and that's the stuff that keeps skin taut. A number of women are most upset by the loss of skin elasticity around their jawline and neck. Sunscreen (look for a broad-spectrum SPF 30 or above) and antioxidants (like vitamins C and E) are your BFFs. Research has shown that estrogen protects against photoaging, so preventing sun damage—a major cause of sagging skin—is especially important as estrogen wanes. Unfortunately, treating sagging at home is tough. In-office, dermatologists turn to devices like Sofwave, Fotona, and Ultherapy to tighten skin noninvasively. Or, for major results, surgeons offer a full-blown menopause makeover.

ACNE: You break out like you're back in puberty. A couple of things are happening. For one, those yo-yoing hormone levels are causing a preponderance of testosterone compared to estrogen (which is diminishing at a faster rate), and that can trigger breakouts, explains Dendy Engelman, MD, a dermatologist in New York City. "Estrogen also assists with keeping cortisol levels in check," she says, "so when estrogen decreases, there's more cortisol to prompt the sebaceous glands to produce excess oil and provoke acne. This is why managing stress to ease up on cortisol is so important for reducing the chances of triggering flare-ups." Engelman is also adamant about wearing sunscreen daily to prevent the acne-irritating inflammation UV exposure causes. For a more targeted solution, she'll prescribe spironolactone, which blocks the androgenic hormonal effects leading to breakouts. As an alternative to meds, there's a noninvasive laser called AviClear, which uses light to suppress the sebaceous glands and prevent excessive oil production to treat mild, moderate, or severe acne. You may also want to add a pro-level exfoliation peel at a dermatologist's office.

“If you find that you have a **doctor** who keeps **gaslighting** you about how you’re **too young to be in perimenopause**—even though you just had a **hot flash** in the waiting room that **popped all the lightbulbs** and **summoned Lucifer**—it is time to **get a new one.**”

—SAMANTHA BEE,
ON HER SHOW HOW TO SURVIVE MENOPAUSE

HAIR ISSUES

It's not your imagination: Hair can become drier, thinner, and frizzier during perimenopause and after menopause. The key players—estrogen and progesterone—affect hair growth cycles, follicle health, and the natural oils that keep strands smooth and shiny. Because estrogen fluctuates during perimenopause, changes aren't linear. "Sometimes your hair may look thicker and healthier; other times it may be thinner and duller," says Debra Lin, PhD, chief scientific officer at *Better Not Younger*. Once you've gone a full year without a menstrual cycle and are officially postmenopausal, some of these changes may be permanent.

Hormone replacement therapy may help slow some of these changes, but topical treatments can also play a role. Audrey Kunin, MD, a dermatologist in Santa Rosa Beach, Florida, recommends 5 percent topical minoxidil for women who are shedding more than 100 hairs per day. Red-light LED therapy has also shown promise in stimulating growth and reversing follicle miniaturization.

Experts agree that scalp care is essential. Keeping it clean, hydrated, and free of buildup reduces inflammation and supports healthier follicles. Lightweight scalp serums with ingredients like niacinamide, ceramides, and caffeine can hydrate without clogging pores. Thickening shampoos with biotin or proteins can make strands feel fuller, while deep conditioners and smoothing treatments help combat dryness and frizz. Supplements may offer additional support, Marmur notes, especially formulas containing B vitamins, vitamins A and C, zinc, and silica—though evidence remains largely anecdotal.

THINNING: A study in the journal *Menopause* found that more than half of postmenopausal women experienced female-pattern hair loss. As estrogen declines, its balance with dihydrotestosterone (DHT)—a hormone linked to hair loss—is disrupted, says Dr. Kunin. Low estrogen can also shorten the hair's growth phase and delay regrowth, while aging follicles produce finer strands, leading to less overall density.

DRYNESS AND DULLNESS: Reduced estrogen lowers sebum production, which normally lubricates the scalp and hair, explains dermatologist Ellen Marmur, MD. Without that oil, the scalp becomes dry and flaky, and strands turn brittle, dull, and prone to breakage. Dryness can also make the scalp more sensitive, weakening the skin barrier and increasing inflammation, especially when thinning leaves the scalp more exposed to environmental stressors.

CHANGING HAIR TEXTURE: "You may suddenly have two textures on one head," says salon owner Katelyn Ellsworth, as hormones can alter follicle shape and turn straight hair wavy or curly.

$6 TO 22 BILLION

The **collateral medical expenses** for older Medicare patients who experience **recurring UTIs**

(SOURCE: GEORGETOWN UNIVERSITY)

FLOODING

There will be blood. So much blood. And clots like you've never seen. Some women we know have described some perimenopause periods as crime-scene-level bleeding. It's also known as flooding, which is exactly what it sounds like. Seemingly out of nowhere, you gush enough blood to wipe out super-plus tampons, pretty undies, black tights, or white trousers. Irregular periods are often the first sign something's starting to change. Periods might come closer together, or you might skip a month. When you don't have a regular cycle and you go longer between periods, you accumulate more of the lining in your uterus, the endometrium, than usual. Eventually, it's going to come out, and it can come out all at once. According to a 2014 study, during perimenopause, 77 percent of women will have at least three episodes of prolonged periods lasting 10 days or more (with at least three of those days involving heavy bleeding). Low-dose birth control pills can minimize and regulate bleeding (though they're not an option if you smoke). Period panties can be helpful, too. But if you're bleeding more often than every three weeks, or if the amount is interfering with your daily life, talk to your doctor about treatment options, including HRT or an IUD with progestin, as well as to rule out other causes, like fibroids, polyps, or certain cancers.

GSM OR VAGINAL DRYNESS

It stands for genitourinary syndrome of menopause, and many people think of it only in terms of vaginal dryness (it replaced the medical term *vaginal atrophy*, thank goodness), but in addition to painful intercourse, its symptoms include urinary urgency and frequent UTIs. "Just like your vaginal tissues start to thin out, your bladder lining also thins and becomes less elastic," explains JoAnn Pinkerton, MD, a professor of obstetrics and gynecology at the University of Virginia Health System.

Left untreated, GSM can get progressively worse. "It's not just about sexual pleasure," says Makeba Williams, MD, an associate professor at Washington University in St. Louis School of Medicine. "I have patients who are unable to sit, ride a bike, who cannot wear pants. It impacts their whole quality of life."

GSM stems from the natural dwindling of estrogen during midlife. From that hormonal slowdown, the mucosa, or vaginal lining, takes a dramatic hit, as does the entire vulva. "In premenopausal times, estrogen brings blood flow to the area, which provides oxygen and nutrients that build that tissue, plumping it up and keeping it moist," explains Suzanne Gilberg-Lenz, MD, an ob-gyn and the author of *Menopause Bootcamp*.

If you are experiencing vaginal dryness, get repeat UTIs, or have begun to feel like you have to pee every six minutes, you're not alone. Somewhere around 50 to 70 percent of women will be affected by GSM. Make an appointment with your ob-gyn or primary care professional. If low estrogen is the culprit, vaginal estrogen is an option for virtually *any* woman.

Research shows that these formulations raise blood estrogen levels very slightly, if at all, and typically keep levels within the same range seen after menopause. This makes it a reasonable option even for women who aren't recommended to take oral contraceptives or hormone therapy, such as women with a history of breast cancer or blood clots, she adds.

There's also no age limit as to when you can start vaginal estrogen. We repeat: NO AGE LIMIT. The right time is "any time you're bothered by vaginal dryness, whether it's because you're having painful sex, or uncomfortable burning or itching, or even frequent UTIs," says Rachel Rubin, MD, a urologist and sexual medicine specialist in Bethesda, Maryland. "I have 95-year-old patients on vaginal estrogen. There's no reason why any woman, at any age, has to suffer when we have such a safe, effective option out there."

55.4%

The number of women **ages 30 to 35** reported already suffering **moderate to severe symptoms** associated with perimenopause.

(SOURCE: UNIVERSITY OF VIRGINIA AND THE FLO WOMEN'S HEALTH APP)

FATIGUE & INSOMNIA

It's the number one menopausal complaint around the world, according to a large global survey. There are many potential causes, ranging from night sweats, stress, and diet to insomnia. Probably the last thing you want to do when you're exhausted is get out every day and exercise, but, however counterintuitive, it does give you energy. Even a short walk helps.

For some of us, in the perimenopause and menopause years, it's not rare to wonder, *Am I ever going to sleep again?* About 40 to 50 percent of women will have sleep problems during the transition, sometimes due to waking up from night sweats but also because of naturally decreasing levels of the hormones estrogen, progesterone, and melatonin. If night sweats are your nemesis, hormone therapy can help. It may also help with other things that may be keeping you on edge at 2:47 a.m.—stress, anxiety, depression, an increased need to urinate at night, and more. Sleep specialists recommend cognitive behavioral therapy (CBT), which includes routines and relaxation techniques. Some women report that melatonin helps, but the research is less clear and many find it does nothing. If you're struggling, sleep hacks will matter like never before (no caffeine past midafternoon, a cool—if not frigid—bedroom, no screens in bed). One last thing: If you turn to alcohol to wind down, unfortunately, this is almost guaranteed to disrupt slumber later in the night, so you might want to see if abstaining helps you get through the night better.

GUT PROBLEMS

A long time ago, in a body far, far less bloated, dinner was a joy. You could eat at 8 p.m., have a glass (okay, two) of wine, maybe dessert, and still rally for a night out. Now? Not so much.

Most midlife women report some form of gastrointestinal distress: In a U.K. study (presented at the 2025 annual meeting of The Menopause Society) of nearly 600 women ages 44 to 73, 94 percent reported new or worsening digestive issues during perimenopause or menopause. Bloating topped the list, followed by constipation, stomach pain, and acid reflux.

When hormone levels fluctuate or fall, your digestion takes a hit in several ways.

A 2023 review published in *Current Nutrition Reports* found that a healthier gut microbiome during menopause was associated with better calcium absorption, improved blood sugar control, and a reduced risk of conditions like osteoporosis and breast cancer.

Your gut needs predictability. Regular meals, movement, and sleep all help digestion stay on track. A Mediterranean-style diet with plenty of protein and fiber supports metabolism and gut health, while strength training helps maintain muscle mass to keep metabolism humming. Fermented foods like yogurt, kefir, sauerkraut, kimchi, miso, and tempeh can help maintain microbial balance and digestion. Other pointers: Drink water throughout the day, try a probiotic, eat slowly, and pay attention to what sets you off. Fried foods and sugary desserts are usual suspects for most women, but even healthy options like onions, broccoli, or beans can bring on the bloat and other gastro upsets.

EVERYTHING SLOWS DOWN. Gut motility—how quickly food moves through your digestive tract—slows, meaning food hangs around longer. The result: bloating, gas, constipation, and of course, weight gain.

MICROBIOME MAYHEM: Your gut bacteria help metabolize and recycle hormones. When estrogen and progesterone dip, the bacteria that perform that job get disrupted, creating a feedback loop that further lowers hormone levels. Low estrogen can also weaken the gut lining and increase inflammation—two big reasons why GI symptoms flare.

BMS BECOME A CRAPSHOOT. During perimenopause, estrogen spikes and dips unpredictably. High estrogen relative to progesterone can speed things up (hello, diarrhea), while low levels of both hormones (later in perimenopause) tend to slow digestion, leading to constipation.

RICH FOODS BETRAY YOU. Foods high in fat or sugar are already notorious for causing inflammation and digestive woes. Combine that with the above-mentioned metabolic and microbial changes to your gut, and rich foods are that much more likely to make you feel awful.

NUTRIENTS LEVELS: One of the quieter effects of perimenopause and menopause is that the body becomes less efficient at holding on to key nutrients. Estrogen influences how we absorb, store, and use vitamins and minerals. As levels fall, deficiencies become more common—not because women suddenly stop eating well, but because the rules change.

CHANGES IN BONE DENSITY

In the first five years after menopause, women lose, on average, 10 percent of their bone density. The primary reason is a sharp drop in estrogen, which is critical for maintaining a strong skeleton.

Ten percent might not sound dramatic, but the consequences are serious. Bones are living tissue, constantly being broken down and rebuilt. "Before menopause, we're building them and breaking them down—it's a nice, even teeter-totter," says Kristi Tough DeSapri, MD, founding physician and director of Bone and Body Women's Health in Illinois.

When breakdown outpaces rebuilding, osteoporosis develops—a condition affecting millions. "Worldwide, it's one fracture every three seconds," Dr. Tough DeSapri notes. Hip fractures are especially dangerous: Among adults over 65, fewer than one-third of men and only about half of women are alive five years after the injury.

Healthy bone resembles a honeycomb, with many small holes. In osteoporosis, those holes enlarge, making bones weaker and more prone to fractures. "Most people think osteoporosis is for women in their 70s or 80s," says Dr. Tough DeSapri. "But it isn't. Women are shocked to learn they have it despite lifelong exercise and adequate calcium and vitamin D."

The good news: There's a lot you can do at any age to protect your bones, and slow or even reverse bone density loss if caught early enough.

GET A BONE DENSITY SCAN EARLY. The Bone Health & Osteoporosis Foundation recommends DXA scans starting at 65 for women, or 50 for those at higher risk. But Dr. Tough DeSapri believes that's often too late. "In my practice, everyone gets a DXA by 40," she says, noting that many women already have osteoporosis by their first scan. Risk factors include early menopause, prior fractures, family history, steroid use, smoking, low BMI, and excessive alcohol intake. DXA scans are quick, painless, and typically repeated every one to two years.

CONSIDER HORMONE REPLACEMENT THERAPY. Estrogen slows bone breakdown and stimulates bone-building cells. HRT is FDA-approved for osteoporosis prevention and can reduce fracture risk, though regular monitoring remains important.

KEEP AN EYE ON RESEARCH ON TESTOSTERONE. A 2025 study in the *Journal of the American Academy of Orthopedic Surgeons* suggests testosterone replacement therapy (TRT) may support bone health and reduce hip fracture risk in older women and men. However, the study was retrospective and did not account for TRT type or dosage, so it cannot prove causation; additionally, TRT is not FDA-approved for women and is rarely covered by insurance. Still, experts note that testosterone may enhance estrogen's bone-building effects, suggesting it could eventually play a supportive role alongside existing hormone therapies.

CHOOSE BONE-BUILDING EXERCISE. Higher-impact and resistance exercises are most effective. Weight lifting, bodyweight movements, running, aerobics, and high-intensity interval training (HIIT) place stress on bones, signaling them to grow stronger.

PRIORITIZE CALCIUM, VITAMIN D, AND PROTEIN. Postmenopausal women should aim for 1,200 mg of calcium daily from food and supplements if needed. Vitamin D (600–800 IU daily) improves calcium absorption. Protein also matters: A 2021 study found that higher intake of protein- and calcium-rich dairy reduced fractures by 33 percent in older adults. Women should aim for 100 grams of protein daily from food and supplements. Once discredited as hype propagated by fitness companies, creatine supplementation has been shown to help build muscle mass, which in turn supports overall bone health.

KNOW YOUR TREATMENT OPTIONS. If diagnosed with osteoporosis, early treatment is crucial. Medications—including bisphosphonates and selective estrogen receptor modulators—can significantly reduce fracture risk.

JOINT & MUSCLE PAIN

Nearly 25 percent of women in the U.S. struggle with chronic pain. And, surprise, surprise, the menopausal transition "seems to make everything worse," says Akiko Okifuji, PhD, a chronic pain researcher and clinical psychologist at the University of Utah Health Pain Management Center. Women with menopause symptoms are nearly twice as likely to be diagnosed with multiple chronic pain conditions such as arthritis and fibromyalgia, per a 2019 study. Estrogen acts on the central nervous system to influence pain perception, says Natalie H. Strand, MD, a professor in the division of pain medicine and director of pain research and neuromodulation at the Mayo Clinic in Arizona. "So if your estrogen levels decline, your pain threshold may also decline," she explains. "Things that weren't painful before can become painful, or if you had pain before, it gets more intense."

Inflammation (often a precursor to pain) can also go up. For example, when the cells in the lining of your knee joint don't receive adequate estrogen, the joint becomes inflamed (so you'll notice swelling), which further breaks down cartilage that's naturally degrading a bit by midlife.

The drop in estrogen during the transition is a significant piece of the puzzle, but a host of other factors can feed a persistent and possibly debilitating pain cycle during this overwhelming time.

Orthopedic surgeon and author of *Unbreakable*, Vonda Wright, MD, has described waking up in her late forties feeling as if she'd been run over—going from training for races to hobbling out of bed. She uses the term *musculoskeletal syndrome* to describe a cluster of symptoms she says are "just as common as hot flashes and wreak even more havoc on a woman's health," yet somehow go underdiagnosed as a symptom of menopause therefore untreated by most practitioners. In her practice, Dr. Wright sees patients with joint pain and stiffness, worsening arthritis, and a spate of minor injuries that even highly athletic women never used to experience. What she's describing, she argues, is not a series of isolated aches but a systemic shift tied to hormonal change.

The loss of bone density is one part of the syndrome (see Changes in Bone Density, page 36), but sarcopenia—muscle loss—is another, and research suggests declining estradiol may play a key role. Estradiol (E2), the primary and most biologically active estrogen before menopause, helps maintain both muscle and bone; after menopause, levels fall sharply and the weaker estrogen estrone (E1) predominates, offering less protection to these tissues. Estrodiol's drop during perimenopause and menopause can lead to joint pain, stiffness, or swelling; the hormone has anti-inflammatory properties and helps maintain joint health. That connection may explain why symptoms can feel sudden to someone entering perimenopause, regardless of their fitness history. Some women suffer pain all over their body—known as arthralgia—and their symptoms, like so many others related to perimenopause and menopause, have often been dismissed as "normal aging." Hormone therapy is approved for the prevention of osteoporosis and may be the next frontier for muscle loss, though more studies are needed.

In the meantime, Dr. Wright wants people to remember one mnemonic: "FACE your Future." F is for *flexibility*, improving joint range of motion, because tendons, ligaments, and muscles tend to get tighter as we age. A is for *aerobic training*. "We know that training with lower heart rate most days coupled with higher intensity sprinting twice a week is the combination that is most metabolically efficient," Wright says. VO2 health, which measures how efficiently your body uses oxygen during exercise, is one of the great predictors of longevity—so consider adding short bursts of exercise (in whatever activity you love—running, rowing, cycling, swimming) where you are truly aerobically spent. C is *carry a load* (a.k.a. weight training). E is *equilibrium*, including balance exercises. "Those things will keep us upright as we age," she says.

"I've been longing to say this out loud. Women are born with *pain built-in*. It's our physical destiny—*period pains*, *sore boobs*, *childbirth*. We carry it within ourselves throughout our lives. *Men don't*. They have to *seek it out*. They invent all these gods and demons so they can feel guilty about things, which is something *we do very well on our own*. And then they *create wars*, so they can feel things and touch each other, and when there aren't any wars, they can play rugby. *We have it all going on in here—inside*. We have pain on a cycle for years and years and years, and then just when you feel you are making peace with it all, what happens? *The menopause comes.* The fucking menopause comes, and it is the *most wonderful fucking thing in the world*. Yes, your entire *pelvic floor crumbles* and you get *fucking hot* and *no one cares*, but then *you're free*. No longer a *slave*, no longer a *machine with parts*. *You're just a person*. In business."

— KRISTEN SCOTT THOMAS,
AS BELINDA IN *FLEABAG*

The Lesser-Known Symptoms

The ones that often fly under the radar.

FERTILITY

Amid all the changes of perimenopause, one thing doesn't change: "I've had quite a few 44-year-olds with surprise pregnancies," says Sarah De La Torre, MD, an ob-gyn in Seattle. "I think some women get more casual about birth control in their 40s, thinking there's no way they could get pregnant."

Indeed, it's rare—groups like the American Society for Reproductive Medicine estimate that, by age 40, a woman's chance is less than 5 percent per cycle—but, surprise, surprise, you still can.

"It's hard for women in perimenopause to keep track of ovulation because their periods begin to become irregular," explains Mary Jane Minkin, MD, a gynecologist at the Yale School of Medicine.

If you want to get pregnant, doctors recommend that you see a fertility specialist right away if you're over the age of 35 and have symptoms of perimenopause, such as irregular periods, hot flashes, or vaginal dryness. (If your periods are regular, and you don't have perimenopausal symptoms, the American Society for Reproductive Medicine advises women between the ages of 35 and 40 to try on their own for six months. Women over the age of 40 will most likely want to get a fertility workup much sooner.)

If you don't want to get pregnant, assume that you still might, says Jewel Kling, MD, MPH, chair of the division of women's health internal medicine at the Mayo Clinic in Scottsdale, Arizona. "I tell my patients that it doesn't matter that they haven't had a period for six months, or for nine months—they need to use some form of birth control," she stresses.

The good news is that many of the hormonal methods of birth control you may use, like the Pill, patch, or IUD, can also help treat symptoms of perimenopause. "Most healthy women in their late 40s or early 50s can safely take a low-dose birth control pill," says Dr. Kling. "Since it provides a steady low dose of estrogen, it will control most, if not all, perimenopausal symptoms, including hot flashes, mood swings, irregular bleeding, and trouble sleeping." She recommends that perimenopausal women without contraindications such as blood clots or a past heart attack or stroke take a monophasic pill, which means it provides a steady hormone level, and that they take it regularly to avoid having a period.

Women in perimenopause who can't safely take estrogen—for example, those with high blood pressure or a history of blood clots—can try the Mirena, a hormonal IUD that releases synthetic progesterone to help both treat and prevent heavy bleeding, advises Dr. Minkin. You can also talk to your doctor about taking the synthetic progesterone-only Pill—known as the minipill—as well. A 2020 review of seven studies published in the journal *Menopause* found that using a transdermal progesterone could help improve hot flashes in perimenopausal women. All of these options also help to prevent pregnancy. At around age 55, "your risk of pregnancy is vanishingly small," says Dr. Kling, at which point you can switch to menopausal hormone therapy.

95%

"When a woman starts **skipping two menstrual periods in a row**, there is a 95% chance her **final menstrual period** will be within the **next four years**."

—DR. JEN GUNTER,
THE MENOPAUSE MANIFESTO

SENSORY OVERLOAD

Your perfectly worn-in jeans feel like you rolled around in sand before putting them on. The overhead lights in your office, which have never been worth noticing, suddenly buzz so loudly you swear there's a wasp hive in the ceiling. And, OMG, when did your partner's breathing get so loud?

Welcome to sensory overload, one of perimenopause's strangest and most sanity-testing symptoms. For some women, it's just one sense (like taste, touch, smell) that goes haywire. For others, everyday life ambushes all five for maximum overwhelm.

Heather Hirsch, MD, a women's health expert and the author of *Unlock Your Menopause Type* and *The Perimenopause Survival Guide*, says she sees it all the time in her practice. "Women will tell me they don't want to travel anymore, they don't want to drive on the highway, they can't stand crowded places," she says. "It's the noise, the people, the heightened sensory input. It's this thing they did a million times before, but now something feels off about it."

Sensory overload isn't an official menopause symptom à la hot flashes and night sweats, and there's not a ton of research on the phenomenon. But Dr. Hirsch says that she experienced it herself and has had many patients over the years complain about sudden sensitivity. "It's basically a lowered threshold to filter lots of different inputs from sensory neurons," she says. (For Dr. Hirsch, she suddenly couldn't stand wearing jewelry: Her earrings were heavy; her rings irritating.)

Dr. Hirsch explains it like this: Estrogen is the referee, and your neurotransmitters—like serotonin and dopamine—are the players. In

"What a woman's body is taking her through is **important information.** It's an important thing to **take up space** in a society, because **half of us are going through this.**"

—MICHELLE OBAMA, TO OPRAH DAILY

this case, our players field all of the sensory input flooding your brain every moment, from what you're looking at on your phone to the chilly breeze on your arm and the taste of your gum. "If the referee just says, 'Well, I'm going to take a break, you guys figure it out yourselves,' things just don't go as smoothly as they normally would," she says. In other words, without estrogen to impose order, the input can get overwhelming for your brain. (It might be extra challenging if you have ADHD or autism, since these conditions also make it harder to process sensory info.)

One way to tell if it's hormone-related, and not something else, is that your symptoms come and go rather than bug you all the time. Sensory sensitivity also shows up during other hormone-driven moments in our lifespan. "We see similar sensory changes in pregnancy and postpartum," says Dr. Hirsch. "Even in the week before your period, when estrogen drops, you might have noticed heightened sensitivity. It's why your husband's chewing suddenly sounds like it's on blast, and you just snap."

There are ways to ease the onslaught:

TRACK YOUR SYMPTOMS. Use a journal or app, logging when sensory overload hits. Look for patterns. This will help you suss out if this is hormonal or something else.

ADJUST YOUR ENVIRONMENT. Little things help. Wear noise-canceling headphones at the grocery store if the sound of fellow shoppers puts you on edge, for example. Dr. Hirsch now travels with a small pouch for her jewelry, so when it starts to feel unbearable, she has a soft place to stash it.

SOOTHE YOUR SKIN. If your sensitivity includes itchy skin or newfound issues with scent, use gentle, fragrance-free, and hypoallergenic moisturizers and soaps. If you can't handle textured fabrics, buy softer, looser clothes (thank you, '90s grunge reboot).

TRY HORMONE THERAPY. Dr. Hirsch uses HRT as both a treatment and a diagnostic tool. "If your symptoms improve with hormone therapy, it confirms they were hormonal," she says. "About two out of three women in my practice find relief with HRT."

And take heart—you won't have to live out your days plugging your nose, covering your ears, or death-staring the stranger whose backpack brushed you at the store. "This is probably more of a perimenopause symptom than a postmenopause symptom," Dr. Hirsch says. "Once you're a couple of years menopausal and hormones stabilize at lower levels, I think it should go away for most women." In other words, you will come back to your senses.

MIGRAINES

The first time it happens, you're sure you're dying: a sudden splitting headache (with a side of severe nausea) that makes light, sound, even thinking unbearable. For an estimated 8 to 13 percent of women, migraines strike for the first time during perimenopause. "I've had patients tell me, 'This is devastating. I can't function for days,'" says Dr. Hirsch, an internist specializing in menopause care and founder of The Collaborative, a concierge medical practice. And if you already get migraines, perimenopause can make them nastier, longer-lasting, and far less predictable.

Experts are still unclear on the exact cause of migraine disorders. In perimenopause, though, three changes collide to make your brain more vulnerable to an attack.

First up: the estrogen fluctuations of perimenopause. A sudden drop in estrogen, especially after a stretch of stability or higher levels, can flip the migraine switch in susceptible women. At the same time, your natural progesterone is quietly disappearing, taking with it the ability to calm the brain. And finally, perimenopause's other symptoms—disrupted sleep, stress, even jaw clenching from night sweats—act as triggers. Add it all together and you have a perfect migraine storm. How do you calm that storm?

Start by ruling out red flags. If it's the worst headache of your life or comes with sudden vision loss, weakness, or trouble speaking, go to the ER. Once emergencies like stroke or aneurysm are off the table, a two-pronged plan is usually best: neurology for migraine-specific tools and a menopause clinician to tackle the hormones, says Dr. Hirsch.

On the neuro side, fast-acting medications like triptans and NSAIDs (nonsteroidal anti-inflammatory drugs, like OTC ibuprofen or naproxen) can help stop or shorten migraines. Preventive treatments, including newer migraine-specific drugs like CGRP (calcitonin gene-related peptide inhibitors), aim to reduce the frequency of attacks.

On the hormone side, the goal is to calm the chaos. Some women do better on extended-cycle birth control (meaning no placebo week when you get your period) to even out hormonal swings, Dr. Hirsch says. Others may benefit from menopause hormone replacement therapy.

One important caveat: Treating migraine with aura (a specific type of migraine that comes with a side of temporary visual changes like blind spots and shimmering spots) requires extra caution because these bring a higher risk of stroke. Therefore, any hormonal approach should be managed by someone who understands both headaches and hormones.

Lifestyle adjustments can help reduce your exposure to triggers, too. Track what seems to set off your attacks in a journal, then see where you can make changes (like prioritizing sleep, eating enough throughout the day to avoid a blood sugar crash, or cutting back on blue light exposure). Supplements like magnesium and riboflavin (vitamin B2) may also help reduce migraine severity and frequency, Dr. Hirsch adds.

After menopause, some women (but not all) see their migraines ease with stabilized hormone levels. With luck you'll be one of them—freeing up headspace for all the other midlife mysteries.

OVER 1.1 BILLION

The **number of women worldwide** expected to be **in menopause** or **postmenopause**

(SOURCE: NATIONAL INSTITUTES OF HEALTH)

RINGING IN THE EAR

Just when you thought perimenopause couldn't make you feel any more unhinged, you start hearing things. A ringing, a hum, a buzz, maybe even a whoosh. You may have tinnitus: hearing a sound that has no external source. Here's what's happening: Over time, the tiny hair cells in your inner ear can be damaged by everything from aging and medications to years of loud music (say, blasting Jagged Little Pill in your Walkman). When these cells can't send clear signals, your brain starts searching for sound—and, not finding it, creates its own.

Hormonal shifts can also be a trigger. "Estrogen and progesterone are thought to have neuroprotective effects," Craig Kasper, AuD, an audiologist who specializes in tinnitus. Without them, your brain becomes more reactive. While tinnitus isn't always curable, it's highly treatable. Start with the basics: consistent sleep, moderate exercise (think walks or yoga, not marathons), and long-exhale breathing to calm your nervous system.

Talk to your doctor or an audiologist who may also recommend the following:

COGNITIVE BEHAVIORAL THERAPY (CBT): the gold standard for breaking the attention-anxiety-tinnitus loop.

LENIRE DEVICE: An FDA-approved device that changes the way the brain handles phantom sounds by providing stimuli to the ear and tongue at the same time and has been shown to reduce symptoms

TINNITUS RETRAINING THERAPY (TRT): A longer-term approach (12 to 18 months) that helps many people adapt by using a combo of counseling and sound therapy.

DRY MOUTH

Menopause can give you a foul mouth, and not just the swearing kind (although there's probably plenty of that too). Foul as in uncomfortably dry with bleeding gums and bad breath. Yes, sudden dental issues are another menopausal symptom no one warned you about.

As with most things meno-related, the drop in estrogen is the key factor. Estrogen plays a crucial role in saliva production and composition. When saliva decreases, your mouth loses a critical line of defense against tooth decay, cavities, gum disease, and bad breath. Reduced estrogen can also cause your jaw bones to shrink, so teeth lose their anchor. As a result, they shift, loosen, or even fall out. It also makes gums recede. Toss in stress-related teeth grinding—yep, another menopause symptom—and you're spending a lot more hours in the dental chair.

But this oral upheaval isn't just a mouth problem; it's a full-body one. "When your gums get inflamed, bacteria can seep into the bloodstream," says Daniel Croley, DMD, a chief dental officer at Delta Dental. Once there, it can spark systemic inflammation and increase your risk of cardiovascular disease, stroke, and even Alzheimer's.

To protect your oral health during this transition: Hydrate frequently to combat dryness. Use alcohol-free mouthwash, which is less drying than formulations with alcohol. Snack on crunchy produce (apples = nature's toothbrush). Keep up with regular brushing, flossing, and dental cleanings.

Some dentists suggest sugar-free gum or probiotic lozenges, which let the brain know that you're getting ready for digestion, so your mouth will produce saliva. There are also special toothpastes and mouthwashes you can talk to your dentist or pharmacist about. For severe cases, your dentist can prescribe medication such as pilocarpine tablets to give your salivary glands a boost.

You might also ask your dentist about salivary testing to check your pH and enzyme levels, which can help identify changes potentially linked to hormonal shifts.

15

The number of minutes in the **online appointment** offered by the **first free menopause hotline** launched by Alloy Health in 2025.

BODY ODOR

You smell like a totally different person. And it's not always great. Blame it on fluctuating hormones, causing a ripple effect on your microbiome (remember, you have a microbiome everywhere—skin, vagina, gut). "Hormones and pH balance shifts, bacteria species and counts shift, and thus, odor shifts," says Suzanne Gilberg-Lenz, MD, author of *Menopause Bootcamp*. At the same time, you're likely sweating more, due to hot flashes and night sweats, building a friendly, nourishing environment for your new bacteria community. And if you're dehydrated, your sweat becomes concentrated, which may produce more potent smells.

You may be tempted to take an extra shower each day, but that would be a mistake. "Don't over-cleanse!" warns Dr. Gilberg-Lenz. "You don't want to use harsh ingredients that get rid of your healthy bacteria. Wash normally." Wear breathable fabrics like cotton, hemp, and linen, so you're not trapping sweat, and drink water. Try tracking your triggers. Identify any patterns by taking note of what you eat, drink, and wear, and how stressed you are when odor hits. Certain foods, especially those high in choline (like liver and eggs) or sulfur (such as onions and garlic), have been shown to affect body odor, particularly when consumed in concentrated forms like garlic powder.

Also, Dr. Gilberg-Lenz emphasizes that you shouldn't panic if you're not loving your new smell—your odor will likely keep shifting along with your hormones.

FROZEN SHOULDER...

Medically speaking, it's known as adhesive capsulitis, but "frozen shoulder" sums it up much better. Because that's exactly what it feels like: a sharp tightness in the shoulder that makes it difficult to do simple things like hook a bra or reach that too-high shelf in the linen closet.

It can happen to anyone and typically comes in midlife—another nickname you might've heard is "50-year-old shoulder"—but menopausal women suffer from frozen shoulder way more because the drop in estrogen increases inflammation. Joint inflammation causes tightness, et voilà: You can no longer lift your tweezers to pluck that pesky chin hair.

Unfortunately, frozen shoulder can last for a year—or even three. But there are solutions. Hormone replacement therapy definitely helps, and at-home treatments like heat packs and anti-inflammatory diets can alleviate some pain.

ME:
I need to do a thing.

...AND FROZEN HIP

"I definitely see hip pain in women over 40," says Jessica Tomazic, MD, a sports and exercise medicine staff physician at Cleveland Clinic. In most cases, it can be treated with medication and physical therapy. But diagnosis can be difficult, since one type of hip pain can masquerade as another. Just ask Joseph Conger (also known as Dr. Joe), a doctor of physical therapy and owner and director of Flying Root Physio in New York City. A patient came in with pain that seemed like classic sciatica, but despite treatment, the pain persisted. One orthopedist, an MRI, more physical therapy, and two courses of steroids later, she felt no better. So Conger and the orthopedist tapped a third expert, a physiatrist specializing in differential diagnosis, who finally suggested the pain might be gluteal tendinopathy—where the tendon tissue in your hips and butt starts to deteriorate or becomes inflamed. After six weeks of a new physical therapy regimen, the woman's pain was gone.

That was the first time Conger saw a patient with gluteal tendinopathy. Since then, he's treated several more women in menopause for it, and recently, patients have started to come in asking about the condition. Data suggests that four times as many women suffer from the condition as men. As for the menopause connection, estrogen is believed to help keep tendons healthy. But as with so many menopause-related issues, this connection hasn't been studied enough yet to prove a definitive link between menopause and gluteal tendinopathy.

Check with your doctor to determine the cause of your pain—it might be sciatica or arthritis. For gluteal tendinopathy, Dr. Tomazic recommends strength training. "Building muscle is probably the most important thing you can do," she says, and that includes your core. "A stronger core can help reduce undue stress on other areas of the lower legs or the lower extremities," she adds.

BODY:

You did a thing yesterday—that's enough things.

(SOURCE: INSTAGRAM)

FOOT PAIN

“Many women come to their appointment saying, ‘I don’t get it. I used to jog, and now it hurts to stand,’” says Suzanne Levine, DPM, a podiatric surgeon at Millennium Podiatry in New York City. Turns out foot pain is one of the lesser-known—but incredibly common—signs of perimenopause or menopause. “I can often look at a woman’s foot and know she’s in menopause,” says Dr. Levine.

When estrogen starts to fluctuate in perimenopause, ligaments loosen, which can contribute to fallen arches, bunions, or plantar fasciitis. Your feet may even grow longer and wider. Bones get more fragile, increasing your risk for stress fractures. And the fat pads under your heels and the balls of your feet—your built-in shock absorbers—thin out. “Many women develop metatarsalgia, which feels like walking on pebbles,” says Dr. Levine. “Or Morton’s neuroma, causing tingling or numbness between the toes.”

Even your skin changes. “Cracked heels are very common,” she says, as plummeting estrogen levels sap collagen levels and dry everything out.

And then there’s the weight gain that often comes with menopause. Each extra pound adds about three pounds of pressure on your already compromised feet.

Fortunately, the fixes are fairly simple. Dr. Levine recommends these below.

CHOOSE SUPPORTIVE STYLES. Look for cushioning, arch support, and wide toe boxes—even in your flats. This doesn’t mean going full orthopedic. Gayle King loves Sneex, celebrities have worn Sole Bliss on the red carpet, and more stylish options are appearing on the market.

ROTATE YOUR SHOES. It also helps to vary heel heights.

TRY AT-HOME RELIEF. Roll a frozen water bottle under your feet, apply anti-inflammatory creams (like topical Voltaren), or massage sore spots.

STRENGTHEN YOUR FEET. Pick up marbles with your toes or do towel scrunches (placing a towel on the floor and using your toes to crumple it up).

SEE A PODIATRIST. “By age 40,” says Dr. Levine, “every woman should have a gait analysis,” an assessment of your posture and movement to identify potential issues. “Small imbalances now become big issues postmenopause.” Some treatment options include custom orthotics and injections of hyaluronic acid (think facial fillers, but for your joints) or poly-l-lactic acid to restore cushioning and reduce pain. Depending on your specific issue, you might also be referred to a physical therapist to get a personalized routine that improves your strength, flexibility, and pain.

ALLERGIES

Your nose won't stop dripping. Your eyes are always watering. And the lotion you've used since the '90s suddenly gives you a rash. No, you're not cursed—it might just be perimenopause.

Many women in midlife develop new sensitivities to things like perfume, detergent, or certain fabrics, says Tania Elliott, MD, a dual internist and allergist. "It's not rare," she says. "I just don't think people necessarily connect the dots."

Researchers may be starting to, however. A few emerging studies have begun exploring a link between menopause and nasal symptoms, though findings are still mixed.

Let's start with a surprise twist: Technically, what you are experiencing isn't allergies. A true allergy triggers your immune system to produce antibodies, which show up on blood or skin tests. "We typically don't see new-onset allergic rhinitis—like an actual pollen allergy—in people over 50," says Elliott. "What we do see is an increase in nonallergic rhinitis and skin sensitivities."

If it isn't an allergen, what's the real culprit of your woes? It's hormones. (Shocker!) During perimenopause, estrogen levels swing dramatically while progesterone steadily declines. Those shifts affect your body in two key ways.

First, hormonal fluctuations can confuse your immune system. At the same time, progesterone—your natural antihistamine—drops off, letting histamine, the chemical responsible for itching, redness, sneezing, and congestion, run wild.

Second, your skin and mucous membranes, like those in your nose, eyes, and mouth, become drier and thinner. Thinner skin makes it easier for irritants to sneak in, and your body may try to compensate for dryness by making your eyes water and your nose leak like a faucet.

This perfect storm of hormonal chaos and immune overreaction makes your body suddenly hypersensitive to things it once tolerated. The result: symptoms that look and feel like allergies, but aren't actually allergies.

If understanding what's happening is the first step; the next is figuring out how to feel better.

TRY ANTIHISTAMINES AND NASAL STEROIDS. These OTC options (like Zyrtec and Allegra) block histamines and reduce inflammation, easing nasal and skin symptoms.

CONSIDER SWITCHING SOAPS, LOTIONS, AND DETERGENTS. Fragrance-free and hypoallergenic formulations can reduce the risk of skin freak-outs.

SUPPORT YOUR IMMUNE SYSTEM. Maintain a healthy weight, reduce stress, and consider probiotics to support your gut, which is a key player in immune health.

TALK TO YOUR DOCTOR ABOUT HORMONE THERAPY. While not a guaranteed fix, it can stabilize the hormonal fluctuations driving these immune shifts, especially if you're experiencing other menopausal symptoms, too.

ANXIETY

Muscle Tension & Aches

BODY ODOR

MEMORY LAPSES

Headaches

VAGINAL DRYNESS

THE 34 SYMPTOMS*

FATIGUE

Electric Shock Sensations

DECREASED LIBIDO

OTHER DIGESTIVE CHANGES

DIZZY SPELLS

BLOATING

Hot Flashes

BREAST SORENESS

IRRITABILITY | **ALLERGIES**

STRESS INCONTINENCE | TINGLING EXTREMITIES

JOINT PAIN | ***Brittle Nails*** | **ITCHINESS**

IRREGULAR PERIODS | **MOOD CHANGES**

OF MENOPAUSE

You're Welcome...

Changes in Taste | DIFFICULTY CONCENTRATING

DEPRESSION | *Osteoporosis*

BURNING MOUTH | **THINNING HAIR**

IRREGULAR HEARTBEAT | SLEEP DISTURBANCE | PANIC DISORDER

NIGHT SWEATS | **WEIGHT GAIN**

***NOTE:** *Not everyone gets every symptom.*

Your Longevity Trajectory

Here's how to harness it for good.

BY JESSIE VAN AMBURG

Living longer seems to be on everyone's mind right now, informing health trends like NAD+ supplementation and protein everything. But for Mary Claire Haver, MD, there's been a population long overlooked in the longevity conversation: the menopausal woman.

"For years, I've been in the trenches with my patients and my community, screaming from the rooftops that midlife and menopause aren't the 'beginning of the end,'" says Dr. Haver, an ob-gyn and certified menopause practitioner. She says that these life stages don't just impact a woman's future years; they're also a "window of opportunity" for intervention. "Education is only half the battle," she says. "Women need access to clinicians who actually understand the science of female aging."

Aging well means we have to look at the body as an interconnected system. Aging well isn't just about managing a hot flash; it's about protecting your bone density, monitoring your cardiovascular risk—which skyrockets after menopause—and maintaining metabolic flexibility. This care is about being proactive and checking the "engine" before it breaks down.

"It's not about the number of years you live," says Dr. Haver. "It's about the quality of those years. Are you strong? Are you sharp? Are you vibrant?"

Dr. Haver admits the fact that women live longer than men is a bit of a biological irony. "We have the 'estrogen advantage' for much of our lives since the hormone provides significant protection for our hearts and brains," she says. "But the "longevity gap" is closing, and while we may live longer, women often spend a greater portion of those later years in poor health compared to men."

The unique challenge for women is the menopause transition. When our estrogen levels drop, we lose that natural protection, which can lead to rapid bone loss and increased inflammation.

The "bro-science" of longevity can be incredibly frustrating because it almost entirely ignores female biology. Women are not just "smaller men." Our hormones, especially the fluctuations of perimenopause, change how we respond to things like prolonged fasting or extreme cold stress .

For women, the most effective biohacks are actually the foundational ones that many of these extreme protocols overlook. Dr. Haver focuses on the "clinical biohacks"—evidence-based interventions like hormone therapy when appropriate, DEXA scans for bone health, and advanced lipid panels. "We filter out the noise and trends to give women what actually works for their bodies and hormones," she says.

Another hidden factor is the connection between menopause and cardiovascular health. Many women don't realize that their risk of heart disease catches up to men's very quickly after menopause. "Proactive longevity care needs to go so much deeper than a standard physical," says Dr. Haver. "We're looking at the things you can't see in the mirror, like your visceral fat and your cardiovascular risk markers, because those are the real predictors of how you'll feel in 10 or 20 years."

Other silent architects of our lifespan include chronic stress. The systemic stress from navigating a world not built for women, including the invisible labor of caregiving, literally weathers the body at a cellular level. This constant cortisol drip leads to premature biological aging and shortened telomeres, says Dr. Haver.

We've all recently heard the perils of social isolation, especially how it can be as damaging to your health as smoking 15 cigarettes a day. For women, a robust community isn't just a "nice to have"; it's a clinical intervention that lowers systemic inflammation and protects the brain. We are also the first generation aging in an environment saturated with endocrine-disrupting chemicals (EDCs). Because our biology is so hormone-driven, especially during the menopause transition, women are uniquely sensitive to these toxins that can accelerate metabolic dysfunction.

Finally, a woman's zip code and education level are often stronger predictors of longevity than her DNA, says Dr. Haver. Access to clean air, nutrient-dense food, and the health literacy to navigate a complex medical system are fundamental longevity interventions.

"The best thing you can do is become an advocate for your own health," says Dr. Haver. Don't accept "You're just getting older" as an answer for feeling suboptimal. Know your numbers, like your cholesterol, blood sugar, and bone density. As she says, "You cannot manage what you do not measure."

what MENOPAU

does MIND

USE

to your

3

The brain you knew is not the brain you've got now

The alarm bells started going off for neuroscientist Roberta Diaz Brinton, PhD, three decades ago, when she saw just how hard women were being hit by Alzheimer's disease. Consider these current stats: Nearly two-thirds of patients diagnosed with the brain disorder are women—a staggering one in five of us will be diagnosed by the time we're 65—and by 2050, as many as 9 million women may end up with the disease. It's even worse for African Americans, who are two to three times as likely as non-Hispanic whites to develop Alzheimer's.

But when Brinton, the director of the Center for Innovation in Brain Science at the University of Arizona, went looking for answers, she found the standard response to these stats unsatisfying at best and maddening at worst. "I kept hearing over and over that it was because women live longer than men," she says. "But we only live about four and a half years longer. That does not explain our twofold greater lifetime risk."

It also doesn't explain why a number of other brain-health issues affect women far more than men: Women are twice as likely as men to develop certain types of brain tumors, nearly twice as likely to deal with depression, and three times as likely to get headaches. We're also much more likely to have a stroke and to develop an autoimmune disorder that affects the brain like multiple sclerosis.

Brinton and a number researchers around the world have begun focusing on what might be going on specifically in women's brains—beyond aging and unlucky genes—to better understand not just what can go wrong, but a more nuanced story. It turns out menopause isn't simply a hormonal decline but a profound neurochemical shift. Estrogen and progesterone, often dismissed as "sex hormones," are also powerful neuromodulators in the brain, directly influencing neurotransmitters like serotonin, dopamine, GABA, and glutamate—chemicals that shape mood, motivation, focus, stress response, and emotional regulation. As these hormones fluctuate and recede, the brain reorganizes itself—sometimes uncomfortably, sometimes dramatically. This "neurochemical storm," as Mindy Pelz, DC, author of *Age Like a Girl*, describes it, can feel destabilizing in the moment, but it may also serve a longer-term purpose: reshaping motivation, priorities, emotional boundaries, and cognitive focus. In other words, the mental turbulence many women experience isn't always a sign that something has gone wrong—it may be evidence that the brain is recalibrating for a new phase of life, one less driven by reproduction and caretaking and more oriented toward discernment, authority, and self-direction.

If some of what happens to the brain during menopause is uncomfortable or even frightening, some of it can feel strangely liberating.

Your Biological Upgrade

Maybe you've seen hundreds of thousands of midlife women joining Melani Sanders's We Do Not Care Club, focused solely on *all the things* they do not care about anymore? There may be scientific and evolutionary reasons for that, says author Mindy Pelz. When estrogen was present, Pelz says, "dopamine, serotonin, acetylcholine, GABA, glutamate, BDNF, oxytocin—you got her girl gang, you got all of them." As estrogen declines, these neurochemicals that once smoothed emotional edges and kept women socially lubricated, decrease, leaving many women feeling raw, exposed, and less able—or willing—to buffer discomfort for others.

This loss of social niceties is often framed as pathology. Pelz disagrees: "Something incredible [happened] to the female brain that rewired itself to make us more built for leadership," she says. The neurochemical changes that feel destabilizing in perimenopause also "lead you to stop caring, stop people-pleasing, stop getting excited about fixing everybody else's problem." Her emphasis is deliberate: "That is by design."

To understand why this "by design" makes sense, Pelz looks to evolutionary biology. Women, she reminds us, spend much of their lives post-fertility. "We live 42.5 percent of our life without a reproductive system," she says. That's not a quirk—it's a clue. The grandmother hypothesis is one framework that helps explain it.

Pelz points to research among the Hadza, a hunter-gatherer tribe in Tanzania, where postmenopausal women—whether or not they are grandmothers—act as vital foragers and knowledge keepers. The men hunt unpredictably, Pelz explains, bringing back food only on rare days. It's the post-reproductive women who reliably gather tubers, watch for threats, and care for children. Beyond sheer survival work, they tell stories—and that matters neurologically. Storytelling activates the hippocampus, a region involved in memory and emotional regulation, and prompts the release of acetylcholine, a neurotransmitter that is vital in brain function, heart and sleep regulation, among other essential physiological activities. In an ancestral context, this wasn't simply a pleasant way to pass the time; it was brain exercise that strengthened cognition and social cohesion.

Women living in modern societies are no longer tribal foragers, but the neurochemical shift that once matched that role still happens. When estrogen declines, the buffering system loosens—and what comes online instead is a brain less tethered to the old social scripts. Pelz points to neuroscience showing that with lower estrogen, the brain becomes more lateralized, meaning women can access focused logical processing without automatically layering in social compliance. The inevitable result is that many women begin thinking first about what they want—a radical departure from a lifetime of culturally reinforced selflessness. (No wonder Sanders's book, *The Official We Do Not Care Club Handbook*, shot to the top of the bestseller lists in its first week on sale.)

Pelz doesn't romanticize the discomfort of menopause or suggest it happens the same way for every woman. What she does offer is a new perspective on this era: Menopause can be the era in our lives when we no longer have the neurochemicals to keep playing by the rules society has set up for us. The shift away from people-pleasing isn't a loss of empathy or warmth; it's the emergence of discernment, clarity, and internal authority—the very traits that would have made post-reproductive women indispensable in human societies and that can allow them to focus a phase of life on what they *do* care about.

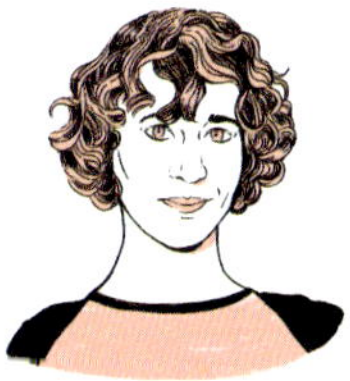

"Maybe midlife crises were just poorly marketed, maybe each one was profound and unique and it was only a few silly men in red convertibles who gave them a bad name."

—MIRANDA JULY,
ALL FOURS

I'm going through perimenopause at the moment. It's really **frying my brain**. It is really **bizarre**, but it is the most **glorious invitation** into a **new season and chapter** in my life... My friend Michaela told me, '**This is an invitation into your wild-woman phase.**'"

—TRACEE ELLIS ROSS,
TO HARPER'S BAZAAR

Rage

You don't know rage until you've felt perimenopausal rage. We're talking red mist. Full-body possession. A sudden, uncontrollable surge that makes you want to drop-kick a decorative bowl across Crate & Barrel because someone had the audacity to brush against you. This Hulk-like behavior has a biological explanation—but hormones alone don't tell the whole story, says psychiatrist Pooja Lakshmin, MD, author of *Real Self-Care*. "There's so much going on at this stage in life—hormonally, neurologically, socially. It's a soup." And many of us are at a boiling point. Hormones spiking, crashing, and ricocheting like the smallest child in a bounce house is definitely one key piece of the midlife rage puzzle: Estrogen fluctuations disrupt serotonin and norepinephrine, both of them mood regulators, leaving you without an emotional buffer. Meanwhile, the drop in progesterone messes with the neurotransmitter GABA, your brain's natural calming system.

The result: miserable, intense anger directed at loved ones, strangers, coworkers, unwashed dishes, randos telling you to "calm down," the person in front of you in the street who is walking way too slowly, that ditzy coworker with the extreme vocal fry, you name it.

Around the same time your brain chemistry is short-circuiting, you may also be deep into a midlife reckoning—the soup's other main ingredient. Maybe your kids need you less. Or your job feels stalled. Or a once-steady relationship has hit the skids.

"There's this feeling of being lost," says Dr. Lakshmin. "Like, I did everything I was supposed to do—I was a good mom, a good worker, a good wife. And now what?"

That disorientation can spark real reflection. Some women make major life changes: a divorce, a new career. Others find a quiet freedom in letting go of who they thought they were supposed to be.

Before you can start interrogating your life choices, you'll need to curb the urge to punch everyone in the face. Dr. Lakshmin recommends considering medical support such as hormone replacement therapy (HRT) or selective serotonin reuptake inhibitors to help get your body back to solid ground. "Once your biology is regulated," she says, "you can start to do the deeper emotional work of figuring out: What's next?" Therapy with a licensed mental health professional can also help you learn healthy coping mechanisms to better process your feelings.

The good news: Even without medical intervention, your hormones will eventually stabilize. According to a 2025 study published in the journal *Menopause*, while anger often spikes in early perimenopause, it tends to fade as you get closer to menopause and emotional regulation improves. In other words, the Hulk inside you will eventually subside, leaving you room to tackle your "why" with the calm precision of Bruce Banner...ideally, without all the ripped shirts.

The Blahs

Did you hit 45 and instead suddenly feel...listless? It might be menopause apathy, an emotional flatness and a lack of motivation that can strike during the hormonal fluctuations of this transition. "Estrogen tends to be energizing for most of us," explains Jessica Nazzaro, DO, an ob-gyn at Cleveland Clinic, menopause expert, and medical advisor to hormone-tracking company Mira. While estrogen levels normally drop off each month before your period, perimenopause causes more frequent low-estrogen spells, so PMS-style exhaustion is a more regular occurrence.

Progesterone also subsides during menopause, Dr. Nazzaro says. This hormone is calming and helps with mood regulation; having less of it can lead to emotional valleys that are challenging to climb out of. (Cue staying home instead of going out with your girlfriends, avoiding your coworkers, and feeling generally unmotivated.)

Cortisol, a.k.a. the stress hormone, is the final piece of the puzzle. "As we age, cortisol doesn't peak as much in the morning," Dr. Nazzaro says; instead, it might spike more throughout the day. Translation: You may struggle to get out of bed in the morning, yet feel activated when you don't actually need it (see 4 p.m. road rage). All of these hormonal factors can conspire to make you feel seriously dull, tired, emotional, and like you just DGAF.

Menopause apathy isn't an official diagnosis; it's more of a description for a common experience. Since it tends to manifest in ways that mirror other physical and mental health issues, Dr. Nazzaro advises women to raise these concerns with their primary care providers. They'll ask you about your relationships, stress levels, sleep, alcohol consumption, and any other circumstances, as well as test levels like iron and vitamin D, to try to understand what's going on. If you rule out other issues, trying hormone replacement therapy can be a solution. "I've had people go on HRT, and then say, 'I feel like myself again. I have energy again. I can get out of bed,'" Dr. Nazzaro says.

Anxiety

For some women, anxiety at midlife shows up as a low-level hum of unease that won't turn off. For others, it arrives as sudden panic, racing thoughts, or a sense that the nervous system is permanently stuck on high alert. It's easy to interpret this as a sign that something is going wrong in the brain. But neuroscientist Wendy Suzuki, PHD, offers a more precise—and less alarming—way to understand what's happening.

First, anxiety itself is not a malfunction. As Suzuki emphasizes, anxiety is "a normal human emotion that is protective." Its role is to keep us alert to danger, risk, and uncertainty. Second, Suzuki suggests a reframing that can be especially useful during this transition: Rather than treating anxiety as a verdict—proof that something is broken—she describes it as information. "On the flip side of your anxiety," she says, "is something that you cherish." Anxiety about health often reflects a deep value for vitality; anxiety about work can signal purpose or responsibility; anxiety about relationships may point to connection that matters. Seen this way, anxiety isn't just noise—it's also data.

So why does anxiety spike in some women in midlife? Estrogen and progesterone support balance among neurotransmitters like serotonin and GABA, which normally help calm fear and stress responses. When that hormonal support wanes in perimenopause, anxiety can feel louder and harder to manage. At the same time, cortisol—the body's primary stress hormone—often runs higher or stays elevated longer during midlife, further amplifying anxious signals.

Add to that disrupted sleep from night sweats or early waking, along with the real pressures many women face at this stage of life—demanding work roles, caregiving for children or aging parents, financial strain—and it becomes clear that menopausal anxiety is rarely driven by a single cause. It's the product of intersecting biological shifts and lived stress, converging on a brain that's being asked to adapt in real time.

While Suzuki is careful not to overstate what science knows about the cause of these symptoms, she notes certain behaviors influence the neurochemistry of the anxious brain. One of the most consistent tools? You won't be surprised to hear it's physical activity. Exercise, she explains, gives the brain "a bubble bath of neurochemicals," including serotonin, dopamine, noradrenaline, and endorphins. Dopamine, in particular, plays a critical role in the prefrontal cortex—the area responsible for focus, emotional regulation, and decision-making—and increasing it can temporarily improve both mood and clarity.

Suzuki doesn't deny that menopausal anxiety can be severe or that it sometimes requires clinical care or prescription medication to help manage. Panic and anxiety disorders are real illnesses, and menopause can unmask or intensify them. For many women, the most important shift isn't eliminating anxiety, but understanding what it's responding to—and learning how to bring the nervous system back into balance.

"I wish that **somebody had told me** that a lot of the **issues** I was going to have in **perimenopause** were going to manifest as things that were **anxiety** or **depression** or **rage.**"

—STACY LONDON,
TO FLOW SPACE

Depression

Depression, a.k.a. anxiety's less frenetic mental health counterpart, can arise in midlife, and a growing body of research suggests that some women might be more biologically vulnerable during this window than others.

First, the timing matters. Large-scale studies now show that perimenopause itself—not postmenopause—is the highest risk period for developing depressive symptoms. A 2024 meta-analysis pooling data from more than 9,000 women found that rates of depression were significantly higher during perimenopause compared with premenopause, while the delta between pre- and postmenopausal depression was negligible. In other words, it's the *transition*—when hormones are fluctuating most—that appears to carry the greatest average risk.

Second, a woman's own mental health history is one of the strongest predictors of depression. Long-running data from the Study of Women's Health Across the Nation (SWAN) show that women who had persistent or higher depressive symptoms earlier in midlife were far more likely to experience depression after their final menstrual period, regardless of other health or social factors. Translation: depression doesn't usually come out of nowhere. Patterns matter.

Family history also plays a role, though not always in the way people expect. Research suggests that having close relatives with depression raises baseline risk overall—but interestingly, the added risk associated with the menopause transition itself may be most visible in women *without* a family history. For women who never saw themselves as depression-prone, perimenopause can be the first time mood symptoms feel unfamiliar and destabilizing.

What's especially important—and actionable—is that depression risk during perimenopause isn't just about hormone levels being "low." Studies show that estradiol variability (how much natural estrogen levels swing up and down) predicts depressive symptoms, particularly in women experiencing high levels of life stress. In other words, hormonal instability plus stress is a potent combination.

Finally, physical symptoms can be early clues. Research has found that women who experience hot flashes or night sweats earlier than expected are significantly more likely to report clinically meaningful depressive symptoms. These symptoms aren't just disruptive to sleep; they may be signals of underlying vulnerability.

In addition to traditional treatments, such as antidepressants, cognitive behavioral therapy, and lifestyle changes, there are a few interesting treatments to consider. "Also, a lot of people are [now] talking about iron in your brain," says Angela Weyand, MD, a pediatric hematologist and associate professor at the University of Michigan. "Because it's a known factor for making things like serotonin and dopamine, which are involved with mood. I am not saying that everyone who has depression just needs iron, but there is probably a subset of patients that, if we corrected their iron, wouldn't even need other things." Dr. Weyand notes that the World Health Organization recommends screening for iron deficiency, and she's seen that women in perimenopause, especially those with heavy periods, can have low levels, as measured by their ferritin levels. Kelly Casperson, MD, author of *The Menopause Moment*, says that a 2018 study published in *JAMA Psychiatry* found that hormone therapy may help ward off symptoms of peri- and postmenopausal depression in some women. Researchers found that only 17 percent of women with the hormone patch developed clinically significant depression, compared with 32 percent of those in the placebo group. As researchers learn more about the biological drivers of depression during perimenopause and menopause, the range of potential treatments is beginning to expand as well.

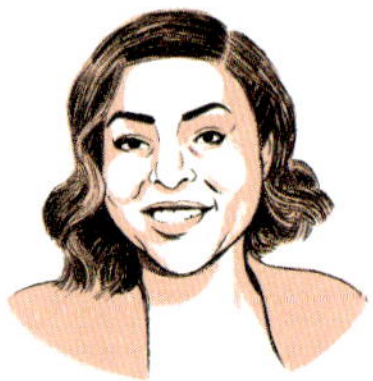

"I would get so low, really, really low, beaten, like never before. You may have those days [when] you're like, 'Oh, I just don't feel like getting out of bed. I just want to sleep in,' but you don't feel heavy. I was just starting to feel heavy a lot...suffocating.... It just came out of nowhere."

—TARAJI P. HENSON,
TO *SELF*

Brain Fog

This one is a biggie. “Up to about half of women report issues with brain fog during menopause,” says Rebecca C. Thurston, PhD, Pittsburgh Foundation chair in Women’s Health and Dementia at the University of Pittsburgh. “They’re wondering, ‘Why can’t I think as well as I used to?’ It’s a common complaint I hear among my patients and research participants. And it’s very distressing.”

“Meno brain” doesn’t manifest in everyone, but for those affected, it’s one of the earliest symptoms to strike. It’s particularly challenging because perimenopause typically sets in around your mid- to late 40s, when many women are nearing the peak of their careers and used to “being at the top of their game cognitively,” Thurston notes.

Although *menopause brain fog* isn’t a scientific term or medical diagnosis, it covers a constellation of symptoms, like difficulty recalling words, names, and numbers; blanking on appointments or events; misplacing common items; and having trouble concentrating or task-switching, among others. “It really represents a change in your own sense of how your brain is functioning,” says Pauline Maki, PhD, director of the Women’s Mental Health Research Program at the University of Illinois at Chicago.

Anecdotally, many women say meno brain has turned them into a spacey, mentally sluggish, barely functioning version of themselves. They may blank on familiar people’s names or forget how to do tasks they’ve mastered for years. “Women are pulled in so many directions,” Thurston says. “We’re so good at multitasking, then all of a sudden, it becomes much more difficult.” Sometimes, these cognitive ripples are so disruptive that they can feel like a harbinger of dementia. These changes are not trivial—it’s embarrassing, humiliating, and even frightening when your mind no longer feels like your own.

When your hormone levels are less like a symphony and more like chaos, the brain responds by getting foggy and having difficulty regulating mood. Some older animal and human studies suggest that estrogen withdrawal can spur changes in the hippocampus, the brain’s memory center, Thurston says. However, experts haven’t established a direct link in humans between a decline in estrogen and a dip in memory function or other aspects of cognition. That’s partly because estrogen is wildly in flux in perimenopause (the hormone’s ebb and flow stabilizes as the transition progresses). “A measure of estrogen on one day might not necessarily be a good measure of the overall hormonal milieu of a woman," says Miriam T. Weber, PhD, an associate professor of neurology and obstetrics and gynecology at the University of Rochester Medical Center in New York.

Maki, who has researched menopause and cognition for 30 years, says she used to think brain fog was simply "an estrogen story," but the overall picture, as she's learned, is more complex. "We know all women go through hormonal changes and eventually lose estrogen," Maki says. "But not all of us experience cognitive changes."

"I couldn't remember what a toe was called the other day. I called it a foot finger."

—*THE CHANGE*, A BRITBOX ORIGINAL COMEDY DRAMA SERIES ABOUT MENOPAUSE

Turns out, other menopause symptoms can play a major role in how foggy you feel, too. Experts say the three biggies are sleep disturbances, mood changes like spikes in depression and anxiety, and hot flashes. Yes, studies have shown that this symptom alone can lead to cognitive strain. "The female brain has to work considerably harder to learn and remember verbal material when hot flashes are involved," Maki says.

While more data is needed, Maki also notes that Black and Hispanic women, particularly those with lower incomes, are more vulnerable to these cognitive changes than white women, in part because women of color are more likely to have severe menopause symptoms and less likely to be properly treated for them. Women who carry a BRCA gene mutation (the biggest genetic risk factor for breast and ovarian cancer) and have their ovaries removed early may also face a higher risk of fogginess for a year or more post-surgery.

While each person's experience is different, brain fog seems to be transient. Many women find that their cognition goes back to baseline postmenopause. The brain likely adapts to its new normal and "appears to rewire itself," Maki notes. More good news: Experts stress that

44–62%

The percent of women in **midlife** and **post-menopausal** women who **report a decline in memory**

(SOURCE: NATIONAL INSTITUTES OF HEALTH)

feeling foggy during menopause does not put you on the fast track for a neurodegenerative disease like Alzheimer's.

That said, taking good care of your brain during midlife ensures it's the most resilient it can be in the years ahead, Maki says. That starts with addressing your other menopause symptoms, since they contribute to brain fog. If you're plagued by hot flashes, hormone therapy is an excellent treatment option. Mental health support (via therapy, medication, or both) can lift depression, chronic stress, and anxiety. For sleep issues, cognitive behavioral therapy for insomnia (also called CBT-I) is the gold-standard method for getting real rest.

Beyond symptom management, everyday habits matter more than most women have been led to believe. Lifestyle changes that have been shown to help brain health? Research suggests that regular physical activity supports brain health by improving blood flow and helping preserve memory and thinking skills as we age. A Mediterranean-style diet has been shown to be associated with better brain health and slower cognitive decline. Meaningful connections with friends, family, and community have been associated with better brain health and a lower risk of cognitive decline.

Dementia

"We know that Alzheimer's disease can take about 20 years to develop prior to a diagnosis and that the average age of an Alzheimer's diagnosis is about 72 to 75," says neuroscientist Roberta Diaz Brinton, PhD. "It doesn't take a rocket scientist to do the math and see that when you subtract 20 from the average age of an Alzheimer's diagnosis, you run into the average age of menopause, which is 51."

Over the past few decades, even more research has provided compelling reasons that women's brains are more vulnerable than men's to certain diseases. "Sex differences in our biologies—different chromosomes and hormones, for example—affect every chronic disease," says Jill Goldstein, MD, a professor of psychiatry and medicine at Harvard Medical School and executive director of the Innovation Center on Sex Differences in Medicine. "So does our gender, including things like social roles and expectations. I am more optimistic than ever that we can have an impact on how we prevent and treat disease if we pay attention to the importance of these differences."

As we've all learned, when it comes to transitions in a woman's life, puberty, pregnancy, and perimenopause are the big ones that play a key role in shaping—and changing—the female brain. And while we may think primarily about reproduction when it

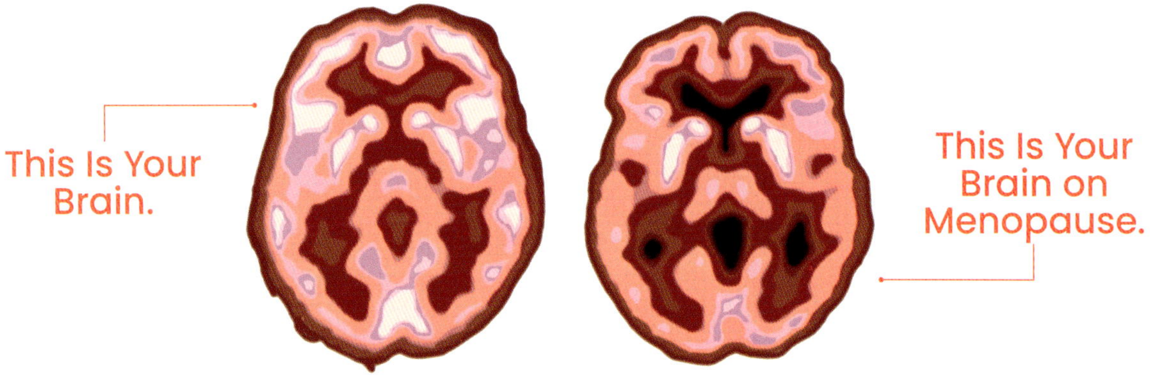

comes to sex hormones, they actually serve a number of functions that have nothing to do with reproduction and everything to do with how the brain uses energy, says Lisa Mosconi, PhD, director of the Alzheimer's Prevention Program at Weill Cornell Medicine/NewYork-Presbyterian and author of *The Menopause Brain*.

"We know that estrogen encourages formation of new connections between brain cells, which makes the brain more resilient and adaptable," says Mosconi. "It's also a neuroprotective hormone that actually shields brain cells from harm." In men, testosterone works in similar ways, helping their brains work optimally.

Yet after men experience a surge in testosterone during puberty, their hormone levels stay relatively steady until andropause, sometimes called male menopause, when those levels gradually decline. (That can happen any time from a man's 40s to his 80s—or never.) Women, on the other hand, go through multiple surges and dips in estrogen, thanks to our menstrual cycles and pregnancy, and we experience a drastic plummet in the years leading up to menopause. "If you consider estrogen as fuel for the brain rather than just for making babies, the magnitude of this dip in estrogen around menopause becomes a lot clearer," says Mosconi.

Changing hormones in the female brain also accelerate the aging process, says Mosconi, weakening our neurons and making our brains more vulnerable to age and disease. For example, when Mosconi looked at brain scans of perimenopausal and postmenopausal women, she found 30 percent reduced brain energy levels. Interestingly, men of the same age showed minimal brain changes or none. Mosconi's and Brinton's research on the differences in how female and male brains metabolize glucose may help explain these findings. "In both men and women, the brain consumes quite a bit

"Dr. Lisa Mosconi is a neuroscientist who is really looking at the female brain during perimenopause, and it's amazing that there have been no real full-scale studies about what happens to the female brain during the time that we start to get these symptoms. And, she actually took images, because she says, 'Okay, here's your brain. Here's your brain in perimenopause.' And they look different. Not only is the structure of your brain changing, but the metabolic activity in your brain is changing. And it's bright when you're premenopausal, and then it just kind of goes dim for a bit. It shrinks." **—SHARON MALONE, MD**

"I can feel the **hormonal shifts** happening, the **sweating**, the **moods**—you're all of a sudden **furious for no reason.**"

—GWYNETH PALTROW,
TO GOOP

of glucose—its primary source of fuel," says Brinton. "But in women, estrogen regulates up to 25 percent of this glucose metabolism." Any condition that limits the brain's ability to either take up glucose from the blood vessels or convert that glucose into energy will have an impact on brain function, Brinton adds. This explains why women often experience cognitive decline when estrogen drops during perimenopause.

Yet something even more alarming starts to happen when having less estrogen slows down your brain's glucose metabolism: Your brain sends out a starvation response. "The good news is that your brain starts pulling peripheral fat from your thighs and belly to get this auxiliary source of fuel to tide you over," says Brinton. "But over the long haul, the brain doesn't like not getting enough glucose—and it will actually start to 'eat' its own white matter for energy." (White matter unites different brain regions into networks that perform various tasks.)

This relatively new understanding of the many ways in which estrogen protects the brain may help explain how male and female brains age differently, says Mosconi. "Generally, 40- to 60-year-old men have high brain energy levels, but for women, there's a marked decline in brain energy during menopause. And for those with a predisposition to Alzheimer's, there tends to be an increased risk of developing Alzheimer's amyloid plaques during menopause. To be clear, not all women develop Alzheimer's plaques, and not all women with the plaques develop dementia. We are working to better understand this risk."

Rather than treating symptoms when we're older, we need to take brain-boosting steps now. Recent population-based studies estimate that over a third of all Alzheimer's cases could be prevented if people made key lifestyle shifts. The best part: It's never too late to start.

If you're looking for a science-backed diet for your brain's health, loading up on veggies, herbs, fish, fruits, nuts, beans, and whole grains (the Mediterranean diet) is the way to go, says Mosconi.

In females younger than 65, physical activity is associated with a 30 percent lower risk of Alzheimer's compared with those who are sedentary, and women age 65 to 70 who exercise see a 20 percent risk reduction. "Not a big fan of the gym?" says Brinton. "Just try to sneak in more movement throughout your day. Even little bouts of lower-intensity movement throughout the day will get your heart rate up and increase blood flow to your brain, which helps to keep it healthy."

"As you get older, you have to build in additional repair and recovery time, which happens while you sleep," says Brinton. So follow the good sleep-hygiene advice you've heard before: Limit screen time at night, establish a relaxing bedtime routine, spend time in natural light to regulate your circadian rhythm, and avoid daytime naps.

Female neuroscientists have just started to study the concept of "cognitive load" (the mental gymnastics most women do to keep all the balls in the air) and its impact on our brains. "Having some mental load is a good thing," says Jessica Caldwell, PhD, a neuropsychologist focused on sex-based brain research, but when this added responsibility gets overwhelming, "you've got a potentially chronic stressor that's really bad for your brain." Be honest about what you can juggle—and what feels like too much.

What Your Mind Can Do to Your Menopause

One woman reflects on the family crisis that rocked her world—and her body—to the core.

BY KIRA VON EICHEL

I knew a woman whose family fled the Soviet Union in 1985, when she was 7. At the train station just before the border, her mother was taken into custody by Soviet guards. In the 24 hours they held her mother, a circle of hair from the child's scalp simply fell out. Her mother was released, they made it to Italy, and by the time they had settled in Baltimore, her hair had grown back. The story always stayed with me. What the fear of losing her mother will do to the child's body in a matter of hours.

In my case, it was the inverse. I was in my early 40s when, out of the blue, we had a very sick child. I didn't lose my hair all at once, but my body changed, almost overnight. We went from being a normal enough family to one in a constant state of crisis. I spent hours every day filling out forms in waiting rooms, arguing with arrogant doctors and insurance companies, pleading with kindly ones, alternating all-night vigils with my husband. I became a desperate comber of articles, medical papers, and blogs. I arranged meetings with friends of friends (of friends) who might have a lead; anything to grab hold of some invisible steering wheel that would give us the illusion of control.

My husband and I were like harried army medics, and as nothing upon nothing worked, the wonderful us we had been just faded into two exhausted housemates who happened to share children. Mounting terror and disagreement slowly calcified into resentment. I tried to keep dates with friends, and if I made it to the appointed place at the appointed time, I tried not to cry. And often failed. The best people stuck around, but many others fell away.

I was also still trying to keep our other child's life humming. School events, volleyball tournaments, birthday parties, appointments, mother-daughter dates. In theory, I was a machine and killing it. And looking back with empathy for that woman in her early 40s, I do see a fierce warrior queen who swam people to shore with one arm tied behind her back. The gift of motherhood is that you believe you can actually lift a car if needed. Even with life sliding quickly from a recognizable path, you tell yourself you will find a solution and you will fix everything for everyone.

But something always gives.

This time it was my body that gave. In spite of a pretty healthy lifestyle, I gained 25 pounds. Parts of my body I'd never thought could expand seemed almost cartoonish as they bulged and stretched. Like puberty on fast-forward, if you added another set of breasts on top of the ones already there. A once thick mane of hair was now diminished, collecting around the shower drain seemingly by the handful with each washing. Every morning I awoke to the imprint of a sweat-drenched body on my sheets, like a chalk outline of a formerly functioning self. At the cocktail parties I dragged myself to, to maintain some semblance of a social life—even as I knew an emergency call would drag me home minutes after arriving—I flushed hot as the earth's iron core from the inside out with the first glass of red wine or if conversation got awkward. "Is it hot in here?" I wondered aloud as I peeled off as many layers as I politely could mid-party. Everything was bone on bone. Noises. People.

Even worse, a once wonderful, fun, close, and happy sex life disappeared. I had always loved men, and most especially the one I'd chosen. Suddenly, I was meh. And so we moved further apart still. It must be stress, I thought. A smart friend wasn't buying it and recommended I get checked for an autoimmune condition or a thyroid issue. After 18 tubes of blood were processed, the answer came back that I was, by the numbers, menopausal.

"But I haven't even experienced perimenopause," I said, somewhat dazed.

When was my last period? (I didn't remember; too busy.) When did your mother experience it? (Later.)

"Usually it tracks," the doctor said. She asked me if there was anything unusual going on. She had a kind, concerned look on her face. I told her the same way I told everyone then. A litany of sad details repeated so often to doctors and specialists that it sounded like a school prayer or a mantra. A series of lines that had come to define us.

She nodded as she kept steady eye contact and told me that extreme stress can accelerate menopause.

I thought of my friend who'd lost her hair when she thought she'd lost her mother. Was my body so on the nose, such a cliché, that any threat to its offspring would flip my reproductive kill switch?

I came home stunned. And a little relieved. After languishing in the soupy, hellish limbo of no real answers or solutions in every other aspect of life, this was, at least, tangible. And by now, I was an expert, PhD-level researcher. I was going to slay menopause, at least. I told my husband almost as an afterthought, with a sort of get-a-load-of-this-style bewilderment.

He barely registered it. "Huh... Funny." And on to putting out the next fire.

That night it occurred to me that this was the end of something. And that I had no clue what the other thing after the something was going to be. For about three days, I fixated on this shift in identity. Who was I without my period?

Would I still be attractive, sexy, juicy?

Was it something to be grieved? All the physical discomfort aside, something felt like it was being wrested from me against my will. The end of fertility felt like the end of me. Or of some secret, special vibrancy accorded me by the slightly miraculous alchemy my body performed each month.

> "I didn't stop existing when I went through menopause unexpectedly early. It's like I got to walk through a secret door."

The Dylan line comes to mind: "Ah, but I was so much older then. I'm younger than that now."

God, I was earnest and misguided. And I took the idea of fertility so seriously, even though I was finished with having kids.

In a way, the ongoing high-stakes juggling act I was engaged in was helpful. I would say that I mourned my idée fixe of my fruitfulness and sexiness for about a minute. I was aware of the thought, and then life just needed me to move on, fast. I did have to deal with the very real symptoms. On top of the body going wonky, I found myself standing in front of my desk, at the bottom of the stairs, in my child's room, rooted in place wondering what I was doing there. Had I filled out this form, returned that call, picked up food? It was like trying to grasp at mist. On the other end of the spectrum, things like the wrong nonorganic milk made me want to stuff my fist in my mouth and scream into the void. The extremes were unbearable bedfellows. They were disruptive and not helping me be the person I needed to be. A true child of the 1970s, I researched and tried every tea and herb and modality out there. Nothing helped enough. I learned Vedic meditation. That helped with a lot of other things. (Thank you, Robert Hammond.) I ate only the good nutritious things. I did yoga. (Thank you, Kula Yoga.) But I was still trying to function with what felt like giant ballasts pulling me below the waterline after each attempt to clear it. And the messaging from the profit-generating world of how to be a better woman was telegraphing that if I only did more, ate less, purchased more powders and creams, I would be in control of my destiny. Finally, after much research about the misleading Women's Health Initiative study from 2002 that scared a generation of women off hormone replacement therapy, and consultation with my doctor, I started bioidentical hormone replacement therapy. The best way to describe what happened once that kicked in is that you could throw a refrigerator at me, and I would catch it, no sweat. Maybe even while holding an inexpert but informed conversation about nuclear fission on the side.

Eventually, I switched to regular hormone replacement therapy—my executive function skills are just too lacking for the bioidentical rigmarole. There was some thinking that we might stimulate my system enough to get it all back.

It never did come back.

But here's the funny thing. Now, at 50 and watching all my close friends get thrown into the spin cycle: what a gift. A release. A deliverance, too. I love being done. I love the benefits of being postmenopausal. Beyond the freedom from the monthly piece. Other things happened. I got calmer. Stronger. Wiser. Less risible. My perspective on people, things, life got longer and kinder.

More important than anything at all: Our kid got better. I know to be grateful for it every single minute of every day. My husband came closer again. We decided to ditch the alienated-housemate thing and remember that we fell in love way back in the early 1990s for some excellent reasons. I'm grateful for that, too. I missed him. The desire came back. More intentional and sweet in the passion.

I also learned that most people are only there for the good times, and they disappear fast in the bad. It sounds like a terrible and awfully disappointing lesson. Ultimately, it wasn't. It makes you absolutely cherish the ones who stick around even when you're faltering and breaking. You end up feeling very rich in human kindness and generosity. Grateful. It's a pretty my-cup-runneth-over feeling.

I didn't stop existing when I went through menopause unexpectedly early. It's like I got to walk through a secret door. I am still a woman, I am still sexual, but a lot of the noise is gone. I am less distracted. By now it's a worn cliché, but you really do care less about what other people think. There's a contentment that grows deeper roots. It isn't a giving up or settling for less, per se. It's an even wilder thing. It opens up whole worlds you'd otherwise never have noticed. Sometimes, when I'm feeling particularly grateful for all this change wrought, that old "Maybe it's Maybelline" ad runs through my head and I picture myself and my brilliant, wise, funny friends looking resplendently our age, gallivanting across a city street, and I replace the tagline with "Maybe it's menopause."

what MENOPA *does to your* RELATIO

USE

4

NSHIPS

If your tolerance, libido, or patience are no longer on speaking terms

Menopause doesn't necessarily announce itself as a relationship problem. But by showing up as bad sleep that becomes irritability, a body that no longer absorbs stress the way it used to, or cognitive changes that make multitasking harder, menopause starts to have a knock-on effect with friends and family. The social arrangements women have been maintaining—at home, at work, in love—often no longer hold.

While menopause does not undermine love or competence, as discussed in the prior chapter, it can decrease our surplus capacity—the ability or urge to smooth over friction, absorb discomfort, and keep going without comment. For many women, that capacity has been central to how relationships functioned. When it diminishes, the change can feel abrupt or even alarming to the people in our lives.

Long-term partners might be dealing with assumptions formed in earlier decades, when the body and mind were maybe a little more forgiving. Dating in midlife brings new intimacy into a body that may feel unfamiliar, unpredictable, or even painful. At home, mothers and daughters can find themselves moving through perimenopause and puberty at the same time—two hormonally intense transitions colliding in close quarters. At work, company expectations remain fixed on uninterrupted productivity, emotional steadiness, and quiet endurance, even as our bodies seem to go rogue every five minutes.

This is why menopause changes relationships even when no one means for it to. It often clearly reveals which social dynamics were built on mutual care and which were quietly subsidized by one person's ability to cope.

The good news is that this moment also comes with unexpected freedoms. When you stop being able to carry everything gracefully, you stop being expected to do so. Conversations get more direct. Boundaries get less theoretical. People who can adapt do; people who can't become easier to identify.

Many women find that the relationships that survive this phase are simpler, more honest, and—surprisingly—lighter. It's also when private frustration starts to feel less private, and the desire to change the conditions around us becomes harder to ignore. Many women find new friend groups or online communities, or join efforts to make positive change in the larger world. What comes next isn't less connection with others, but more closeness, more honesty, more ease. Here are seven relationships that may change at midlife.

With Your Spouse

Can menopause cause a crisis in a marriage? When Oprah Daily teamed up with menopause practitioner and ob-gyn Mary Claire Haver, MD, and posed this question to her patient list, hundreds of women shared stories of how menopause strained or even upended their marriages. Sometimes, the beginning of the change marked the end of the relationship; other times, hormone replacement therapy (HRT) or couples counseling saved it. Some couples came out the other side stronger than before, and one woman's menopause journey culminated in her feeling "as alive and vibrant as a teenager"—who quite emphatically did not want to be married.

According to a 2022 survey by the Family Law Menopause Project in the U.K., 73 percent of women blamed menopause for their divorce. Dr. Haver says she can see why: "The reasons are multifactorial. It may simply be that menopause gives her enough clarity to realize, *It's okay for me to go. I need to focus on me.* Other times, it's mental health changes that are not being addressed—in perimenopause, we see a surge of depression and anxiety, which can take a tremendous toll on relationships. I hear a lot about menopausal rage, too, when women are just yelling at their loved ones all the time, and they can't pull themselves out of it." The final piece of the jigsaw? Changes in libido that come with the transition, as well as physiological factors that can make sex downright painful. "It's a huge problem—95 percent of women have a loss of interest in sexual activity," Dr. Haver adds. "There's definitely a hormonal issue there, because the hormones that tell our brains that sex is a good idea dramatically change during menopause. That leads a woman to be less likely to be interested in sex, even when she loves her partner."

Psychiatrist and researcher Judith Joseph, MD, agrees that the link between menopause and the breakdown of relationships is inextricable: "While many people don't want to pathologize menopause, we need to be very realistic and not dismissive of what we're hearing," she says. "It causes changes in the brain that impact mood, sleep, and thinking, and then all of these things impact your identity. With menopause, you're getting challenged on both fronts: Emotionally, you may be more irritable or anxious, and then physically, it might be more challenging to connect with your partner."

Dr. Haver, who is also the author of *The New Menopause*, recommends avoiding making major changes while still in the throes of symptoms. "Something I say to my patients is, 'We need to get you back into you. We need to normalize what's going on with your hormones, so we can get you back in a headspace to be making these huge decisions.' Until you feel like you can function fully, it's probably not a good idea to make major life changes. Divorce may be the best thing for you, but let's get your mind back first. Let's get you sleeping at night and out of this fight-or-flight feeling."

Treatment might help. "Two years ago, my husband asked me for a divorce," says one woman who responded to the initial call. "I finally decided to try HRT. Within two months, my relationship with my husband improved. Now a year and a half later, we're so happy. Menopause could have ruined my marriage. Learning the truth about menopause care saved it."

You also need to communicate what's happening to you—no partner, however empathetic, can be expected to guess.

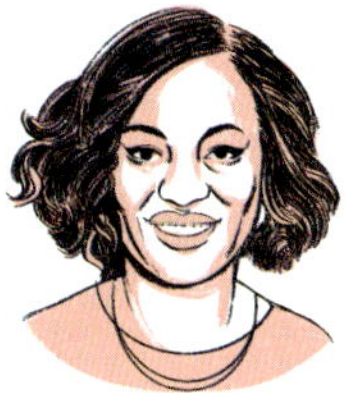

"Menopause is a dark hole, okay? That's what menopause is. And that's where I'm at right now. So I either will love my husband today or kill him today."

—VIOLA DAVIS,
ON *JIMMY KIMMEL LIVE!*

Dear Partner, This Is What Menopause Feels Like

A letter to your better half.

Dear Partner,

I am writing to you because it's time for us to take a trip to the mini med school that is menopause. Sometimes it may seem like the woman you've known all these years is gone, or changed into someone totally unfamiliar. I get it. Sometimes I feel the same way. I've never gone through menopause before, and since it can be different for every woman, I have no idea what to expect. Some days, I feel like I'm going to get through it no problem, and other days, I feel...well, like I won't. Put simply, I feel like I'm springing leaks of symptoms from literally all angles. One day, it might be my mood, mind, memory, or ability to focus. I've been feeling more stress, anxiety, and moodiness than I did when I was a teenager. The next day, my symptoms travel down my body and may involve breast tenderness, bloating, midsection weight gain (even though I haven't changed what I am eating), fatigue, irregular bleeding, hot flashes, and what feels like the ultimate insult—vaginal dryness. Between tender breasts, a bloated belly, and a dry vagina, can you understand why I may not be in the mood for sex?

I want my old self back. I want my "old," younger vagina back! Part of me is afraid that the premenopausal me may be gone forever, and that I may not like the postmenopausal me—and that you may not like her, either. It can be overwhelming.

Part of me is afraid that the premenopausal me may be gone forever.

The thing about menopause is that it's not just about the physical or psychological changes—though those certainly aren't a walk in the park. Society has a stigma against many things pertaining to women, and this is no different. When a man ages, he becomes more distinguished. When a woman ages, she is "past her prime" or seen as less relevant. In the past, even the medical community turned its back on us when we needed them most. Thankfully, that is changing. Doctors are listening and helping, and you can, too. It won't always be this way; I know I will come out of this stage and be better than ever. For now, I ask you to understand that some of these hormonal changes are tough—just like they can be tough during puberty or during and after pregnancy. I will get through it. We will get through it. And by the way, if manopause were a thing, I'd totally be there for you, too.

-Warmly (and I mean that literally),
Your Person

I didn't ever **hate my spouse**, but there were times where I was like, **'Get away from me. I don't want sex. I don't have anything to do with that.** I have **no interest** in talking to you right now.'"

—TAMSEN FADAL,
TO OPRAH DAILY

With Sex

"I have two women sitting right next to each other in a focus group," recalled Melissa Melby, PhD, a medical anthropologist at the University of Delaware. "One says, 'Menopause is great. It means I can have sex with my husband and not worry about getting pregnant anymore.' Her friend laughs. And she's like, 'To me, menopause means I never have to have sex with my husband again.' For both of them, there was this sense of freedom, but for the exact opposite reason."

Melby's point is that as the ovaries start closing down, it's a different story for every woman depending on her physiology, her health, what's going on in her life, the culture she lives in (Melby's focus group was in Japan). And "freedom" is not always the first thing that comes to mind.

"Women tell me their vagina feels like it's shrinking. They're right; it actually is," says Lauren Streicher, MD, author of *Slip Sliding Away*. As mentioned in chapter 2, a lot of physiological changes are occurring: "The vaginal rugae, accordion-like folds that help the vagina expand, become flattened and less flexible. The labia may also diminish. As a result, sex can become painful. It may not just be stabbing and burning. Multiple studies show that often women also experience a loss of libido and have trouble orgasming."

The technical term for what's happening is GSM, genitourinary syndrome of menopause. With advancements in medical science and a better understanding of women's health, experts have strategies that can bring enormous relief.

Topical vaginal estrogen therapy can be a life changer. "Vaginal estrogen, or vaginal hormones, are safe for everybody," says Suzanne Gilberg-Lenz, MD, who's frustrated that the message is still slow to permeate the wider culture. "I repeat, they are safe for everybody, no matter what else is going on." Creams, tablets, and rings can all be prescribed to replenish local estrogen levels, significantly improving vaginal elasticity and moisture. You can use them whether or not

2.9%

Researchers seeking to examine the association between **sexual regularity** and **vulvovaginal-related problematic menopause symptoms** in a 2025 study found **less than 3%** of the participants reported using **vaginal estrogen**.

(SOURCE: MENOPAUSE, THE JOURNAL OF THE *MENOPAUSE* SOCIETY).

you're on HRT. "You're putting those hormones back into the tissue, helping it behave as it did premenopause," she explains.

One suppository Dr. Gilberg-Lenz particularly loves, called Prasterone, is actually DHEA (dehydroepiandrosterone), a hormone that converts into estrogen and testosterone. Talk to your doctor about getting an Rx that works best for you.

You might also start a skin regimen for your vulva that begins with cleansing properly. "Warm water is all you need—seriously," says Dr. Gilberg-Lenz. "No wipes, harsh cleansers, or soap, which will dry you out even more." Next, if you want to turn to nonprescription moisturizers to keep the area hydrated, Dr. Gilberg-Lenz recommends ones containing hyaluronic acid (her favorite moisturizing ingredient) to support that delicate tissue. According to both experts, this alone can make a world of difference in your day-to-day comfort.

Another option is to try technology. Although they're an investment and you'll have to get over the concept of a powerful device being pointed at your private parts, a dermatologist may suggest energy-based therapies to reinvigorate your vagina, according to Dr. Gilberg-Lenz. There are lasers (like the MonaLisa Touch) and radio frequency devices with or without microneedling (like Viveve, Votiva, EMFemme 360, and ThermiVa). All of these options micro-damage the skin, which spurs the body to bump up collagen and repair the tissue in a stronger, more robust way, Dr. Gilberg-Lenz explains, adding that they work best in combination with topical hormones that further enhance healing.

With sex, experts say the use-it-or-lose-it principle is very real, and lubricant makes a huge impact in ensuring pleasure and eliminating agony. "Silicone-based lubes that decrease friction are best because they don't absorb too quickly," says Dr. Gilberg-Lenz. "In contrast, water-based products can actually pull moisture out of the tissue and cause more dryness." She's a big fan of Überlube; its gentle formulation is compatible with sensitive tissues, but it's still durable. Another good option: Replens Silky Smooth Personal Lubricant. Play around with different products to see what works best for you.

Because symptoms and desire change differently for everyone, libido is usually shaped by a mix of hormones, relationship dynamics, stress, body image, and lifelong attitudes toward sex—none of which operate alone. The advice for improving sex in perimenopause and menopause is mostly the same as at other times: Take pressure off performance, expand sex beyond intercourse, talk about it outside the bedroom, schedule time for connection, and make sure sleep, pain, and other health issues are being addressed. Redefining sex as a menu rather than a single act also creates more room for pleasure, intimacy, and connection, especially when spontaneous desire is unreliable but responsive desire is still very much alive. And while it may feel awkward at first, naming menopause and its effects out loud—with partners and clinicians alike—often turns confusion into collaboration, which is one of the most reliable aphrodisiacs there is at midlife.

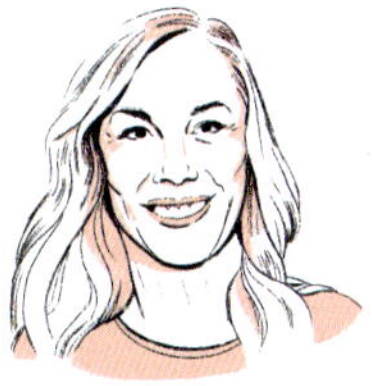

"These boys that are my age... they've laid in the bed next to a woman and thought, 'Is that steam coming off her?'"

—LEANNE MORGAN,
IN HER *I'M EVERY WOMAN* SPECIAL

With the Internet

"The Internet brought my fellow Gen Xers together in new ways," writes Dr. Gilberg-Lenz. "Like so many others, I found community and engaged with experts and regular folks in unprecedented ways. The scale of impact and engagement over the past several years—and the amplification of these messages over social media—cannot be overstated. We saw and heard our stories over and over in both the most intimate and public settings. We finally felt seen and understood." She is not alone. For many women, the Internet and social media have become something different during perimenopause and menopause. What once functioned mainly as entertainment or distraction quietly turns into support. You go online looking for one thing—an explanation for why your heart is racing at 3 a.m.—and realize other people are already there, talking about the exact thing you didn't know how to name. Though as with all things Internet or social media-related, it's about identifying credible experts, voices, medical institutions, and brands to avoid the pitfalls of bad information.

This shift can be especially meaningful for women who feel out of sync with the people around them. Maybe you had your kids closer to 40, and now you're the oldest classroom parent by a decade. Maybe your family culture doesn't allow you to talk openly about bodies, aging, or anything that sounds like a complaint. Maybe your friends are busy, partnered, or simply not here yet. Online, you find shorthand. You find recognition. You find the oddly comforting moment of realizing that symptom—yes, that one too—is part of the picture.

At its worst, the Web can be...well, you know. But at its best, a digital community can be a godsend: a place for practical health information (ideally from reputable sources, and followed up with actual clinicians), shared language, and low-stakes humor. The jokes matter. So does the relief of being seen without having to explain yourself from scratch. The Internet doesn't replace care or connection in real life—but for many women, it's where both begin to feel possible again.

"For us, *midlife is bigger than aging*... By force or by choice, WDNC members have *stopped caring* about being perfect, being liked, being small, or fitting in. We have started caring about *being honest*. We want to *feel how we feel*, *rest* when we need rest, *be messy* when we want to be messy, and be *seen as we are*.... That's what this club is about, and that's *who we are*."

—MELANI SANDERS,
THE OFFICIAL WE DO NOT CARE CLUB HANDBOOK

With Your Daughter

They call it the puberty of midlife, but what happens when a perimenopausal woman shares a house with a daughter going through actual puberty? "Whoever designed it so that women would be going through perimenopause while raising teenagers should be sent a strongly worded letter," actress Katherine Heigl told *Business Insider.* "It's really difficult. Their hormones are all over the place, they're trying to adapt and get used to their new bodies and their new ways of thinking, and I am too. So the only thing I can do is look at them and go, 'Well, at least we're in it together.'" That comparison—menopause as midlife puberty—rings true because the parallels are unmistakable. Both stages bring sweeping hormonal shifts that affect mood, sleep, skin, energy, and self-confidence. Bodies begin to feel unfamiliar. Emotions arrive suddenly and with force. The difference, of course, is experience. You've been through puberty once before; she hasn't. You have perspective, language, and hindsight. She has intensity, immediacy, and the conviction that this version of herself is permanent.

And still, your carefully gathered wisdom lands about as well as your own mother's advice once landed with you. Some lessons simply can't be absorbed secondhand—they have to be felt in real time. There's also the quieter reckoning that comes with watching her move through it. You see her as she is now—young, dewy, luminous in ways she can't yet recognize—and it's impossible not to feel the contrast. Not envy, exactly, but an awareness sharpened by proximity: She has so much ahead of her, while you are firmly in the middle of things. You're no longer unfolding; you're reckoning, integrating, letting go. Holding space for her insecurity and self-doubt can sting, because from where you stand, she is already whole. And at the same time, her youth reflects back something harder to avoid—that you're not glowy in the same way anymore, and the future no longer stretches endlessly outward. It's a tender, disorienting realization, made sharper by love.

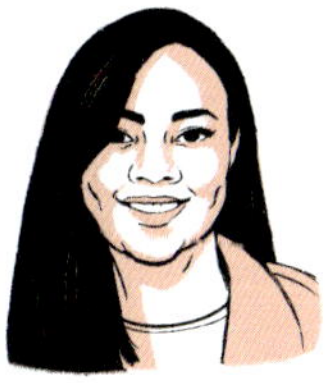

"I'm a human being and something is going on. And we need all to be very cognizant about that and compassionate with ourselves and other people."

—GABRIELLE UNION,
ON *THE DREW BARRYMORE SHOW*

With Yourself

Is there a more pervasive symptom of perimenopause than "I just don't feel like myself"? That phrase comes up again and again in midlife, but rather than signaling what's been lost, this uneasiness can function as a prompt, nudging women to consider: If I'm no longer who I used to be, who can I choose to be now? Many women realize they care less about keeping the peace and more about telling the truth—to others but especially to themselves. They develop a new awareness of limits. They may start to see, clearly and sometimes abruptly, how much time and energy they actually have and how carefully they want to spend it. This can affect relationships, including marriages (it takes honesty to sort out what's a temporary hormonal shift versus what's been quietly wrong for a long time). It can redirect career goals—long hours in a buzzy industry might be traded for a straight-up 9 to 5. It can lead to less time spent with acquaintances and more with ride-or-die friends. Which is all to say, this period enables a kind of truer sense of purpose than prior phases. In that sense, menopause can be less an ending than a reset—one that makes room for a more honest, self-directed version of life.

“I was lucky to be surrounded by **supportive colleagues and friends.** They’ll grab me my bedazzled fan during a hot flash, **breathe with me** while I’m anxious, or just **laugh through it.**”

—NIECY NASH-BETTS,
TO FLOW SPACE

With Work

Did you see this headline? "Women Always Had Hot Flashes at Work. Now They're Done Hiding Menopause." In this *Los Angeles Times* article, a senior lawyer described her deep appreciation when a colleague saw her suffering from a hot flash and presented her with a pretty folding fan. Hot flashes are but one of dozens of disruptions—brain fog, headaches, anxiety, erratic periods, and urinary tract infections, among them—women experience on the road to menopause that can last for as long as a decade.

A fan? Seriously? Surface level and short-term interventions rarely meet the needs of most menopausal employees. Still, it's progress that the term "menopause-friendly workplace" is even being used. Other good news: According to the health care consultancy firm Mercer, 15 percent of large employers in the United States said they would offer or planned to offer some kind of menopause support in 2024, up from just 4 percent in 2022.

The need is growing, too. One in every five employees in the United States is at or close to the other side of menopause, showing up to work while potentially managing great strain on their bodies and brains. A 2023 Bank of America report, Break Through the Stigma: Menopause in the Workplace, found that more than half of the women surveyed said menopause had a negative impact on their work life. And there's massive financial fallout, too: The Mayo Clinic calculated that symptoms like hot flashes, cognitive difficulties, and mood swings cost an estimated $1.8 billion in lost wages per year.

Moreover, the irony isn't lost on us that menopause arrives just as many of us are catching our professional stride. The prime age of women in the U.S. workforce reached an all-time high in 2023. The average age at which women assume top roles in executive leadership? Fifty-four. Mind you, there is still paltry representation in the highest ranks of corporate America: Women hold a mere 10.4 percent of CEO positions in Fortune 500 companies. Managing menopause in the workplace is only one of myriad inequities to overcome. Regardless of their level, losing women at their prime because of the absence of supportive practices and policies impacts productivity and revenue/the bottom line in every industry.

"I have often reflected on my own working-through-menopause story," explains one woman. "The times when my periods were so heavy that I had to max out on overnight maxi pads and still couldn't sit at my desk for more than 30 minutes before having to dash to the restroom and change. The times I lost my temper, lost my train of thought, lost documents that I literally forgot to click 'save' on. It never occurred to me that the experience would have been infinitely more manageable if workplace accommodations were the baseline. And not just a lifesaver for me but also for my colleagues and every single person who relied on me."

There are accommodations still to be made, but if we've learned anything from the pandemic, it is that the ways we work can be far more elastic and inclusive—something that disability advocates have asserted for years. For menopause, the recommendations are simple and concrete: provision of paid health-first (not just "sick") days and consideration of the physical conditions and cadence of the workday (tweaked as needed for things like temperature controls, dress codes, and timing and frequency of bathroom, meal, and beverage breaks). Companies should offer access to menopause-specific health care professionals and medical benefits. Also abundant educational resources for all employees about the mechanics of menopause and a separate, more granular "what to expect" set for those who are directly impacted. Extra credit for targeted materials that address the demands of particular professions: What matters to retail workers might look different for round-the-clock direct-service providers, or for women who sit at a desk versus ones who stand in front of a classroom.

The conversations are just beginning, but the hope is that in the not-too-distant future women in midlife will have a better and more equitable relationship with work.

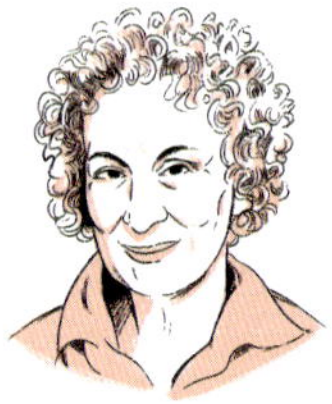

"Menopause. A pause while you reconsider men."

—MARGARET ATWOOD, *WILDERNESS TIPS*

With Your Legislators

Midlife women are suddenly discovering that legislators are people they want to be in touch with, not just during election season. Rhode Island made headlines in July 2025, by becoming the first U.S. state to explicitly ban menopause discrimination and require reasonable workplace accommodations for symptoms like hot flashes and night sweats, adding menopause to its fair-employment protections alongside pregnancy and childbirth. Meanwhile, states including California (where legislation would mandate menopause training and coverage), Illinois and Louisiana (which have expanded insurance coverage for menopause care), and several others have passed menopause-related laws or training requirements, and more than a dozen states have introduced bills on menopause awareness, care, clinician education, and workplace support.

On the federal level, there's still work to do. The We're Addressing the Realities of Menopause (WARM) Act would add public awareness about menopause and related conditions to the Public Health Service Act, and the Menopause Research and Equity Act would require the NIH to evaluate ongoing research and identify gaps in understanding and treatment—but neither bill has passed yet. Menopause may turn out to be the phase of life when women know not only who their reps are but have their offices on speed-dial.

5

what if you **CAN'T FIGURE** *it out*

Trouble–shooting menopause challenges

While some women facing perimenopause and menopause have little awareness about what may be involved beyond hot flashes, others are not starting from zero. They've read the articles, followed the advice, and tried everything from supplements to lifestyle changes to prescription options—yet the relief they were promised never fully arrived, or it faded too quickly.

If you're one of them, this doesn't mean you've failed, you waited too long, or you'll simply have to live with it. More often, this just means the strategies you were offered didn't fully address what was happening in your body, they weren't tailored closely enough to your specific symptoms and stage of life, or no one explained what else could be tried if the first approach fell short.

When this happens, it's not just disappointing—it's exhausting. After a few rounds of trial and error, many women reach a point where pursuing another appointment, another recommendation, or another experiment feels like more effort than they can reasonably take on. Not to mention how challenging it can be to find a health care practitioner who knows their stuff or to deal with insurance companies or find a way to pay for all these treatments. When your days are already overfull, it makes sense that following up on symptoms falls to the bottom of the list.

This section is for women who know something still isn't right—and want a little guidance on how to move beyond the initial options toward approaches that are clearer and more individualized and may bring real relief.

You Were Told Nothing Could Help in Perimenopause

You're not alone. A few years ago, Drew Barrymore sat onstage with Oprah Winfrey, Gayle King, and several doctors taping Oprah's "The Life You Want" series on menopause. Drew, who'd famously experienced her first hot flash on national television while interviewing Jennifer Aniston, said she'd been feeling "dead inside." She was 48, confused, and unsure of what to do next. "I've heard different answers from different doctors," she said. For instance, she was told that there was nothing she could do while she was still getting her period. (Which, for the record, is not true!)

So many women get frustrated when they can't find solutions, says Lauren A. Tetenbaum, LCSW, a therapist and the author of *Millennial Menopause*. Unfortunately, managing the menopause transition is "an ongoing adventure that requires patience and proactivity," she says. "My generation is now navigating the fluctuations—the zone of chaos. I work with my clients on focusing on the present moment. 'What is bothering you the most right now? How can we address it?'"

For many women, though, trying to address even one thing is frustrating. "A lot of people are being told by physicians that perimenopause is just trending right now," says Tamsen Fadal, a menopause advocate and the author of *How to Menopause*. "Women

75%

When researchers from Yale University looked at over **500,000 insurance claims** from women in **various stages of menopause,** they found that **300,000** of the claims were related to patients seeking medical assistance for **significant menopausal symptoms**—and that **75% of the patients left without treatment.**

—**DR. MARY CLAIRE HAVER,**
THE NEW MENOPAUSE

tell me, 'My doctor says, "Not *everything* is perimenopause."'" And while that's true, Fadal says, certain symptoms are related to this phase of life: "If you have 10 hot flashes a day, you need to go talk to somebody. You have severe anxiety, you need to go talk to somebody. You have heart palpitations, you need to go talk to somebody."

There are options: Perimenopausal women might have luck with lifestyle changes or can go on birth control. If that doesn't help, their practitioner might suggest low-dose hormone therapy—or share nonhormonal treatments. "I don't want women to feel like because they are in this stage," says Fadal, "that they have to wait until this deadline 12 months after their last period to get help."

Your Hormone Therapy Didn't Work

"Whenever someone comes to me saying, 'I've tried HRT. It didn't work for me,' I'm thinking about three things," says Heather Hirsch, MD, the author of *The Perimenopause Survival Guide*. The first is the formulation, meaning there are different versions of HRT using different hormones, and this might not be the right one for them. The second is the dose, meaning how much they're taking. The third is the route, meaning are they getting HRT orally or transdermally? (Dr. Hirsch notes that timing is a fourth item to consider, though not as important as these three.)

Let's break it down.

PROGESTERONE INTOLERANCE AND OTHER FORMULATION ISSUES

"There is no one-size-fits-all in hormone therapy," says Dr. Hirsch. "For every woman who comes in and says, 'This changed my life!' there are others who say, 'This stuff's horrible.'" For example, she discovered that about one third of her patients were irritated by progesterone (they felt bloated, sluggish, uncomfortable), which led her to coin the term "progesterone intolerance." Dr. Hirsch found the problem can be solved by prescribing other formulations, including synthetic progestin, or by using an IUD. "You know how they say with 10 digits, you can make, like, trillions of phone numbers?" she says. "It is the same thing with HRT." This is why with new patients, Dr. Hirsch begins by stacking hormones—typically two weeks on progesterone to ensure there are no unbearable side effects, then adding estrogen for two weeks to determine if that causes any issues. If there are, she tries alternatives that may be better for that individual.

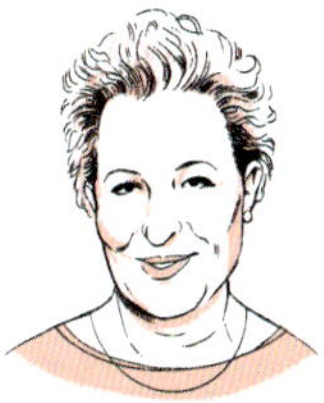

"[Menopause is] all these out-of-body experiences...the real you is over there watching while your body moves in space. Then you go online and have menopausal chats with other women who are having out-of-body experiences."

—BETTE MIDLER,
TO *O, THE OPRAH MAGAZINE*

TOO HIGH (OR LOW) A DOSE

Early on, Dr. Hirsch found that a lot of patients who came to her for a second opinion were on a dose that was too low. "Lately, they're too high," she says. "I'm actually bringing people down and they feel better." She says a few signs that estrogen might be too high are if patients report feeling weepy or have breast tenderness or bleeding.

THE WRONG ROUTE

Dr. Hirsch says many patients default to the patch, but that may not be the best option. She recently met one woman who'd been on the patch for about two years. She wasn't feeling great, and her doctor kept increasing the dose. When Dr. Hirsch tested her levels, it was clear the woman was not absorbing the hormones through her skin. *Menopause*, the journal of the Menopause Society, published a study in 2024 that found "up to 20 percent of women are poor absorbers of transdermal estradiol." These patients might consider oral estrogen for better results.

Your Hormone Therapy Didn't Fix Your Libido or Energy Struggles

Let's say that thanks to hormone therapy, your hot flashes are gone, your joint pain is better, and your night sweats have eased. Vaginal estrogen has helped with symptoms of GSM. Your blood work shows estrogen and progesterone levels in a healthy range.

And yet—something still feels off.

Many women describe feeling "flat," "gray," or disconnected from themselves. Motivation is low. Libido hasn't returned. Workouts don't deliver the payoff they once did. These women are functioning but not thriving. According to menopause specialist Kelly Casperson, MD, a urologist and author of *The Menopause Moment*, this might be the time to consider testosterone, as the hormone is linked not only to sex drive but also to musculoskeletal health and cognitive function. Dr. Casperson says there is resistance to it: Many patients see it as a so-called "male" hormone, but as she explains, "Ovaries make testosterone—this *is* a female hormone." Other patients have only heard of it in terms of treating low libido. But it's more than that: Dr. Casperson says for some women, testosterone can help restore cognitive energy, motivation, and a sense of self in a way that estrogen alone sometimes doesn't. "Many women on testosterone will say things like 'I don't hit a wall at 3 p.m.' or 'I want to finish this project I had put on the side.'" Dr. Casperson has also testified to Congress about its safety—including pointing out that three countries have approved female-dose testosterone. While there is currently no FDA-approved testosterone treatment for women, health care practitioners can prescribe it in low doses off-label for libido issues. Just expect to pay out of pocket, since off-label meds typically aren't covered by insurance.

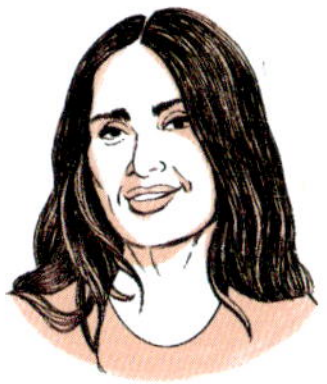

"What we're saying is that there is no expiration date for women—that has to go because you can kick ass at any age, you can hold your own at any age."

—SALMA HAYEK,
ON *RED TABLE TALK*

Hormone Therapy Worked... and Then It Didn't

Tamsen Fadal, author of *How to Menopause*, had success with hormone therapy. A huge relief. "But 18 months later, I started having hot flashes again—I couldn't sleep anymore. I was anxious all over again," she says. "And I was like, 'What the hell?! How did this happen?!'" She went back to her doctor, who, because Fadal was postmenopausal, ran a blood test to check her estrogen levels. (After menopause, the levels don't fluctuate as they do in perimenopause.) The doctor changed her HRT dosage accordingly. Fadal explains that as we age, hormone levels may shift and what worked before may no longer, but health care professionals may be able to find a better protocol. "Now I have a *really* big patch," she says with a laugh.

You Can't Take Hormone Therapy

Many doctors advise women not to take HRT if they are survivors of estrogen-dependent cancers, like some breast and uterine cancers, which use estrogen to develop and grow. (In other words, HRT could help cancer regain its foothold.) Women with a history of blood clots, stroke, or significant heart disease or liver disease are also not candidates for HRT. Other women simply don't want to use hormones. To help these women and their health care providers understand their options, the Menopause Society updated its recommendations for evidence-based nonhormonal management of vasomotor symptoms (VMS, a.k.a. hot flashes and night sweats). The position statement, released in June 2023, includes recommendations for prescription and nonprescription therapies, plus a rundown of treatments that the organization does not recommend due to a lack of supporting evidence (those include acupuncture, herbal supplements, and yoga). These options made their yes list:

PRESCRIPTION MEDS

For decades, hormonal therapy, which reduces hot flash symptoms by roughly 90 percent, was the only FDA-approved treatment for VMS. That changed in 2013 when Brisdelle became the first FDA-approved nonhormonal treatment for moderate to severe VMS—and again in 2023 with another option (see chapter 2 for even more recently approved alternatives). "Everybody's jumping into this hot flash treatment," says Stephanie Faubion, MD, the director of Mayo Clinic's Center for Women's Health and medical director for the Menopause Society. The latest newcomer is elinzanetant, which the FDA approved to treat moderate to severe hot flashes. The drug blocks not one but two brain receptors controlling body temperature. It became available in the U.S. under the brand name Lynkuet in November 2025. The list price for a 30-day supply is $625, but eligible patients with insurance could pay $25 if they get their prescription filled through the digital pharmacy BlinkRx. Other medications for hot flashes are prescribed off-label. Some of those on the Menopause Society's list are gabapentin (an anticonvulsant and nerve pain medication), oxybutynin (approved to treat overactive bladder), and a few antidepressants: venlafaxine (Effexor XR), citalopram (Celexa), and escitalopram (Lexapro).

CLINICAL HYPNOSIS

One study, funded by the National Institutes of Health and done in collaboration with Baylor University, aimed to determine the efficacy of self-administered hypnosis for the issue. Every day for five weeks, patients spent about 15 minutes listening to audio recordings that first helped them relax into a hypnotic state and then had them visualize walking down a mountain path on a cool day or sitting near a lake feeling a cool breeze. The results, published in late 2025, align with those of a 2013 study that examined practitioner-delivered hypnosis for hot flashes. "Across studies, the results have been very consistent," says Gary Elkins, PhD, a professor of psychology and neuroscience, director of the Mind-Body Medicine Research Lab at Baylor, and the research lead on both studies. "This specific hypnotherapy intervention for hot flashes results in a 70 percent decrease in the frequency and severity of hot flashes at the end of a five-week program," Elkins says. "We believe that as hot flashes go away, the hypothalamus begins to regulate normally again."

COGNITIVE BEHAVIORAL THERAPY (CBT)

Another recommended nonmedical approach, CBT works to make hot flashes less bothersome. "The basic idea of CBT is that thoughts and emotions are related, so the focus is on coping with the symptoms," says Elkins, who teaches CBT at Baylor. For instance, if you feel a tsunami of heat coming on, you might begin to panic and think, *Oh no, I'm about to start sweating in front of everyone!* CBT teaches you how to catch the thought, pause, and manage the stress you feel about it with breathing or other exercises. Neither hypnosis nor CBT has side effects, and both can be used alone or in combination with other therapies, including HRT. The only downside has been finding practitioners, but fortunately, research shows that both treatments can be effective when self-directed.

40% & 10%

Up to **40% of women in their 60s** and **10% to 15% in their 70s** continue to have **hot flashes.**

(SOURCE: *CONTEMPORARY OB/GYN*)

You Think You're Allergic to HRT

"I get tons of messages" from women who get a big red mark where their patch is, says Tamsen Fadal, author of *How to Menopause*, and it bothers them. Fadal says the women are not likely "allergic" to hormone therapy, but they may have a sensitivity to the glue on the patch. Changing to a different delivery format—gel, cream, or spray—seems to solve the issue.

You're Still Experiencing *[Fill in the Blank]*

"Menopause can accelerate aging-related changes, but not everything that happens in midlife is hormonal," says Jessica Shepherd, MD, an ob-gyn and the author of *Generation M*. The issue, she says, is that menopause has become a kind of catchall diagnosis. Bloating? Must be hormones. Fatigue? Hormones again. Joint pain? Same. In reality, aging and menopause overlap—but they're not the same thing.

Take gut health, for example. Dr. Shepherd says bloating, gas, and food sensitivity are among the most common complaints she sees—and they're often misattributed to menopause alone. "As we age, our gut microbiome changes, the intestine becomes more permeable, and digestion just isn't as efficient," she says. "That can cause bloating and discomfort even when hormones are well managed." In those cases, hormone therapy might not fix the problem—but dietary shifts (including fiber intake) and microbiome support may. This distinction matters because when women assume everything is menopause-related, they may overlook other fixable contributors. "It's important to step back and ask what else is going on in the body," Dr. Shepherd notes. That includes changes in metabolism, muscle mass, sleep quality, stress levels, and digestion—all of which evolve with age, regardless of reproductive status.

The goal isn't to minimize menopause, Dr. Shepherd emphasizes—it's to broaden the lens. Understanding what isn't hormonal can be just as empowering as treating what is.

Heather Hirsch, MD, the author of *The Perimenopause Survival Guide*, agrees. "If a patient feels like we've done a lot of different adjustments and they're still not 70 to 80 percent better," she says, then it's time to think of what else may help. Like other experts, Dr. Hirsch believes lifestyle choices should be a part of any treatment plan: "If a patient's joint aches and pains don't get better but everything else gets so much better, then I think, 'Okay, maybe it's time we work you up for osteoarthritis.'"

When women separate menopause symptoms from aging-related changes, they're more likely to get the right kind of help—and stop feeling as if their body is failing them for no reason.

“I may not be **as strong** or **as supple** or **as smooth** as in my youth, but I am **comfortable** with my vulnerabilities, **conscious** of my weaknesses, **proud** of my strengths.”

—PAULINA PORIZKOVA,
ON INSTAGRAM

You've Done All of the Above and Yet...

You're suddenly fatigued. Or you're gaining weight. Or you're still mired in brain fog. You've tried HRT, plus lifestyle changes—improving diet, adding weight-bearing exercises, following sleep hygiene practices. Try looking at another common midlife factor: new medications. Many women start or change prescriptions in their 40s and 50s—often for good reasons—but some drugs can quietly mimic or worsen menopause symptoms. For instance, statins can cause fatigue and sleep problems. Some corticosteroids, diabetes medications, and antidepressants can cause weight gain.

Mental health medications can further complicate the picture. SSRIs and SNRIs, prescribed for anxiety or depression that came on in midlife, have helped so many women. But they can cause symptoms women assume are hormonal. SSRIs and SNRIs can cause hot flashes, night sweats, and fatigue, but it's trickier than it appears: The same medication that causes hot flashes in one woman can improve them in another. For instance, venlafaxine (an SNRI with the brand name Effexor) is an effective nonhormonal treatment to reduce hot flashes. "That's what makes this so confusing," says Harita Raja, MD, a psychiatrist who specializes in women's mental health. If you've started a new prescription, a full medication review might reveal why you still don't feel like yourself and what you might want to adjust next.

You Were Told PCOS Would Go Away in Menopause

If you've been diagnosed with polycystic ovary syndrome (PCOS), you're one of approximately 8 to 13 percent of women globally who have spent their reproductive lives dealing with a constellation of difficult symptoms, such as irregular cycles, weight gain, painful periods, cystic acne, and excess hair growth. Because PCOS impacts ovulation, women with the condition might think of menopause as the victorious finish line for all of the issues and anguish it doles out. No more fertility, no more problems, right? Wrong. Doctors and researchers are just beginning to learn how PCOS plays out in menopause and beyond, and what women who suffer from it should keep an eye out for. Here's the breakdown:

LINGERING INSULIN RESISTANCE

This is common among women who struggle with PCOS during their reproductive years, but it can also last into menopause. When your cells resist insulin, your blood glucose levels can rise. Over time, this phenomenon leads to weight gain, type 2 diabetes, and metabolic syndrome (a group of several disorders related to weight gain that can lead to heart problems and diabetes). According to a study in *Gynecological and Reproductive Endocrinology & Metabolism* that examined how insulin resistance affects women in menopause, women with PCOS typically have abundant estrogen without enough progesterone. Couple this with the cortisol boost that comes with aging and you have a recipe for worsened insulin resistance as you progress through menopause. Consider asking your doctor to check your A1C (a test that measures your average blood sugar levels over three months) and your current glucose levels. Mary Jane Minkin, MD, a clinical professor of obstetrics, gynecology, and reproductive sciences at Yale School of Medicine, says women with PCOS should behave much as diabetes patients do: monitoring blood sugar, sticking to a good diet (she recommends—surprise!—the Mediterranean diet), and getting in as much aerobic and strength training as you can. If your glucose levels are high, an endocrinologist can help you explore possible treatment options, such as metformin, a commonly used diabetes medication that decreases insulin levels, or drugs like Wegovy and Ozempic for weight loss. Also noteworthy: Researchers in the study found that women in perimenopause who used transdermal hormone replacement therapy appeared to be protected from weight fluctuations.

HIGHER RISK OF COGNITIVE DECLINE

While menopause is notorious for messing with your memory, women with PCOS might receive an added blow: A longitudinal study published in *Neurology* revealed a link between PCOS and cognitive dysfunction later in life. Kaitlin Casaletto, PhD, an associate professor at the University of California, San Francisco's Weill Institute for Neurosciences, who helped conduct the study, says women who met the criteria for PCOS showed worse cognitive performance at midlife (ages 48 to 60) than women who didn't. "This suggests that the endocrine, cardiovascular, metabolic, and other differences associated with PCOS are risk factors for brain health," she explains. "Our data may also suggest PCOS influences brain vascular function, which is known to change with age and is associated with age-related cognitive changes." Casaletto says a diet high in vegetables, whole grains, and legumes is associated with a 30 percent reduced risk of stroke and cognitive decline. Referring to the brain as "elastic," she recommends staying active and social, getting enough sleep, and staying curious, like learning a new hobby or language or talking to someone new.

"I miss the thought of having lil babies in my belly and periods and womb stuff like that. **BUT I AM NOW ABLE TO SHARE MY WISDOM AND JOYFULLY GROW INTO THE GLITTER DRIPPING PHOENIX CREATED THRU THE FIRE.**"

—ERYKAH BADU,
ON INSTAGRAM

POTENTIAL FOR DEPRESSION

Numerous studies have linked PCOS with an increased likelihood of depression. Though researchers are still working to determine precisely why, it's likely something of a vicious cycle related to insulin resistance—impaired insulin signaling can impact your mood, and your mood can also cause behaviors that lead to resistance. As Casaletto's study notes, all those fluctuating hormones that can cause depression in women with PCOS worsen in menopause. If you notice a downswing in your mood or just feel inexplicably blah, tell your doctor and consider consulting with a therapist or psychiatrist for further evaluation.

INCREASED RISK OF HEART DISEASE

Women with PCOS could be at a 30 to 40 percent increased risk of developing cardiovascular disease during pregnancy or later in life. Erin Michos, MD, a professor of medicine in the division of cardiology at Johns Hopkins School of Medicine, has worked on several studies examining the connection between PCOS and cardiovascular disease. Most adult sufferers of PCOS should "get a comprehensive cardiovascular screening; have their blood pressure, glucose, and lipids checked; make sure they know their A1C; and try to maintain a healthy weight to offset some of these risks," Dr. Michos says. She also recommends a low-dose CT scan called a coronary artery calcium test, which can identify calcified plaque in the heart arteries. Your cardiologist can order it, but be sure to check and make sure your insurance covers it.

You Remain Exhausted

It's the number one menopausal complaint around the world, according to a large global survey. And there are a number of potential causes, including lack of sleep, stress, and diet. But if you've ruled those out *and* remain brain-dead, bone-weary, please-don't-ask-me-to-move exhausted *and* your doctor says your thyroid, hemoglobin, blood pressure, and cholesterol tests all came back normal, you might want to check one more thing, says Angela Weyand, MD, a pediatric hematologist and associate professor at the University of Michigan.

One of Dr. Weyand's clinical interests is iron deficiency, whose symptoms include extreme fatigue, weakness, headaches, light-headedness, cold hands and feet, and "unusual cravings" like chewing ice. Iron deficiency is often overlooked because it's commonly equated with anemia, the most extreme stage. A hemoglobin test can tell you if you're anemic, but it doesn't measure iron itself.

Ferritin, which reflects how much iron the body is storing, may be a better indicator. But there's no consensus on what's "normal." The World Health Organization's healthy range is from 15 to 150 µg/L, yet lab definitions of normal vary widely. Dr. Weyand notes that these ranges are based on supposedly healthy women—many of whom are iron-deficient themselves. So if you're at the low end, it's worth a conversation about treating it.

This is especially relevant for women in perimenopause, who may suffer from irregular and heavy menstrual bleeding, which puts them at increased risk for iron deficiency. In addition, symptoms of iron deficiency (things like fatigue, mental fog, insomnia, mood changes) can overlap with symptoms of perimenopause. The International Federation of Gynecology and Obstetrics recommends iron-specific screening (ferritin) in all women starting at menarche and for the rest of their lives.

Conventional wisdom suggests postmenopausal women shouldn't have iron issues because they no longer menstruate. But if someone's ferritin has hovered around 11 to 15 µg/L for decades and stays there, they may still feel wrung-out, freezing, lightheaded, and exhausted—technically normal but still unwell in the earlier years of menopause. With patients in perimenopause or early menopause, doctors are often concerned that low iron levels might signal internal bleeding or colon cancer; they are also reluctant to suggest supplements because iron overload can damage organs. So screening matters, Dr. Weyand says, but so does listening to symptoms.

The good news: Iron deficiency is treatable with supplements or, in some cases, iron infusions administered by IV. And when Dr. Weyand's patients finally get what they need? "I feel like a new person," they often tell her.

Deema Tabbara Lopez
@prettyonfridays

Perimenopause tip:

To feel better, just exercise six times a day, eat 600 grams of protein, lift heavy, meditate upside down, drink moon-charged water, take 78 supplements, and do eight cartwheels around your house every hour.

Easy. Why are you crying?

Your Doctor Doesn't Get It

There's no one-size-fits-all in menopause care. The right provider depends on how you like to communicate, what you want beyond prescriptions, and what your budget (and insurance) will cover. As some women have learned the hard way, not every ob-gyn has expertise in the menopause transition. You can find a list of health care providers certified by the Menopause Society (formerly the North American Menopause Society or NAMS) on its website. Many menopause specialists suggest an in-person appointment, because doctors can run tests and offer hands-on care right away. That said, we've heard from many women that doctors with that expertise often have long waiting lists for an appointment. We also know that in many areas, virtual visits are the only option. A few things to think about below.

WHO'S PROVIDING CARE

The right expertise can make all the difference, so look for clinicians with menopause-specific training or Menopause Society certification. Our experts suggest calling the office and asking if the practitioner has experience treating menopausal patients and the training to prescribe menopausal hormone therapy. Also consider: Do you want a long-term relationship with one provider or are you okay with a team-based approach?

HOW YOU WANT TO COMMUNICATE

Do you like in-person visits or face-to-face video visits, or would you rather message on your own schedule?

Questions to Ask Your Doctor

Help your health care provider help you.

To get the most out of your appointment, take a few moments to prepare. Start by asking yourself what it is you want to accomplish. Do you want to know if you can still get pregnant? Are you looking to alleviate your symptoms? Something else entirely? Whatever your goal, have one in mind before you get to the reception desk.

JOT DOWN SOME NOTES

You're used to whipping out your phone the moment you enter an exam room so you can answer the perennial doctor's office question: When was your last period? But you'll need to be prepared with a bit more info when discussing perimenopause and menopause. This means tracking your periods and/or documenting your symptoms, including what they are, how often they occur, and how bothersome they are.

PREPARE A LIST OF QUESTIONS

Writing them on a piece of paper, or in the notes section of your phone, can help you remember what to discuss and keep the conversation on point. Here are some questions you might want to ask.

- ☐ Are the symptoms I am experiencing within the normal spectrum?
- ☐ How do I know if the symptoms I'm having are because of menopause or something else? What tests do you recommend?
- ☐ What can I do to alleviate my symptoms with the fewest possible side effects? What should I do if that doesn't work?
- ☐ Are there any natural products that can help?
- ☐ Can I still get pregnant? What do you recommend using for birth control at this stage of menopause?
- ☐ What should I know about the next stage of menopause? How can I prepare?
- ☐ What's not normal? When should I call or come back?
- ☐ What can I do to protect my bone health throughout menopause? What other steps should I take for my overall health?
- ☐ Do I still need to have regular Pap tests and breast exams?
- ☐ Don't leave out the intimate details.
- ☐ If your concerns include anything having to do with sexual function, whether vaginal dryness, painful sex, or low libido, don't hesitate to bring them up. After all, sexual health is part of your physical health.

Online Menopause

	ALLOY HEALTH	WINONA	STELLA (BY VIRA HEALTH)
THE PROMISE	One-Time Fee + Unlimited Access	Community + No Consultation Fees	Comprehensive Care
WHAT SETS IT APART	Your doc responds within 24 to 48 hours, and there's no appointment juggling or additional consultation fees. Just don't expect face time with your practitioner—it's a text-only relationship.	For those who just want a prescription, Winona charges you only for the actual medication—no appointment costs, no monthly memberships. A doctor reviews your info and approves you within hours, then you get your treatments delivered directly. It offers both FDA-approved and custom-compounded options to treat your symptoms.	For those who are looking for more than a prescription refill. You'll see the same provider (a doc or nurse practitioner) for video visits (typically available within a week), and your care continues between appointments through the companion app.
BEYOND HRT	The company started with hormone therapy but expanded to support other midlife health needs, such as sex, weight management, and skin care. It offers both FDA-approved and custom-compounded treatments (including estrogen-infused moisturizers and serums), plus community support groups and educational webinars.	With 34,000-plus women in its community app, as well as nearly 29,000 in its Facebook group—not to mention regular free, in-person meetups nationwide—Winona also provides the support network many women crave during this transition. It also hosts virtual live doctor Q&As, and some brand ambassadors host book clubs in their communities.	A year's access includes unlimited one-on-one wellness coaching, habit tracking, and educational resources. With live Q&As and webinars, you'll feel supported through the whole process.

Care

From messaging-only plans to full-service virtual clinics...

MIDI HEALTH	EVERNOW	MYMENOPAUSERX	PANDIA HEALTH
Training Depth + Scale	Research-Backed Flexibility	Speed + Quality Control	Messaging-Only Simplicity
What sets Midi apart is its rigorous provider training and extremely thorough offerings. Every clinician completes more than 50 courses in midlife women's health and continues with weekly education to stay current.	Can't decide between video calls and messaging? Evernow offers both. You can book insurance-covered video visits or choose an unlimited-messaging membership.	Need help now? MyMenopauseRx typically offers video appointments within 48 hours—no endless waiting while your symptoms spiral. Your care will be managed by a clinical team, all certified by the Menopause Society, with a supervising menopause-certified doctor reviewing all notes to make sure nothing gets missed.	For those who hate phone calls, Pandia makes menopause care as easy as texting, with doctors who typically reply within two business days. The platform's approach is straightforward: Address the essentials—hot flashes, night sweats, vaginal health, and bone strength—with FDA-approved treatments.
Care is delivered through video visits with the same provider over time, building continuity and trust. Midi's clinicians include nurse practitioners (NPs), certified nurse-midwives (CNMs), doctors (MDs), and naturopathic doctors (NDs) who specialize in women's midlife health. All treatment is overseen by menopause doctors who collaborate closely with clinicians to create a personalized care plan for every patient.	The company is flexible about treatment too: FDA-approved meds can be sent to your local pharmacy (insurance applies) or delivered directly to your home; in some cases, custom-compounded prescriptions may be available. The app keeps everything in one place—symptom tracking; lifestyle programs for sleep, nutrition, and strength training; and direct access to your provider.	Beyond HRT, the company covers the full spectrum of the menopause experience—from hair loss to bone health and mental health changes—and prescriptions can be sent to any pharmacy the patient chooses. There is also a community page that allows patients to interact with one another and offers education, such as a course on pelvic floor health.	Pandia also offers invite-only live events with its doctors to answer FAQs or discuss hot (sorry) topics.

You Can't Figure Out How to Pay for Treatments

If you were a middle-aged man suffering from erectile dysfunction, you could walk into a neighborhood pharmacy and buy a 30-day supply of sildenafil (the generic version of Viagra) for about nine bucks out of pocket, and no, that's not the insurance copay. That's the basic cash cost with a coupon.

A menopausal woman in search of affordable estrogen, however—a requirement not just for her sexual health but for her overall health and well-being—might spend hundreds, if not thousands, of dollars on it per year. Urologist Kelly Casperson, MD, author of *The Menopause Moment*, finds the whole estrogen racket both infuriating and confusing to her, too. Though she is a well-informed doctor with excellent health insurance, her local pharmacy recently tried to charge her a $265 copay for generic estradiol cream, a local vaginal estrogen treatment. "I know enough," she says, "because I prescribe this every day, that I pulled up my GoodRx app, typed in the pharmacy, and it was $28. I showed them that and said, 'I wanna pay the $28 cash price.' They said, 'Yep, no problem.'"

You might use Dr. Casperson's strategy at your pharmacy or you might try an online telemedicine start-up. Joanna Strober, Midi's cofounder and CEO, says, "The visits are usually covered by insurance, although there is also a self-pay option. When covered by insurance, the cost varies based on the insurance copayment and the deductible, but most women pay less than $40 for their visit." Strober says an estradiol patch, a systemic estrogen treatment, is their most popular choice, and they can usually work with insurance companies to get the copay for that down to around $15 to $20 a month. They will also work with your insurance to get the cost of progestin down to $10 per month. But again, this depends on your policy.

For people with bare-bones, state-sponsored health insurance and a giant deductible, it might make more sense to pay out of pocket, though it can be hard to navigate this nontransparent

4

"There are **four distinct patterns** of **vasomotor symptoms** among women in North America.... This means there's approximately a **25% chance hot flushes** will be **minimal or nonexistent**, a **25% chance** of being a **super flusher**, and a **50% chance** of falling **somewhere in between.**"

—DR. JEN GUNTER,
THE MENOPAUSE MANIFESTO

system. Billionaire entrepreneur Mark Cuban understands this—it's why he started Cost Plus Drugs, to offer "safe, affordable medicines with transparent prices." He realized he could be a health care activist and turn a respectable profit at the same time. "Women's health is a specific focus of CostPlusDrugs.com," says Cuban, whose company also sells affordable birth control. "We consider it critically important to provide as many branded and generic medications dedicated to women as we can."

The cash prices of generic drugs on Cost Plus are often lower than an insurance copay for the exact same medication. How? Cuban purchases generic medicines in bulk directly from the manufacturer, cutting out the middlemen. Then he marks up the cost of each drug by 15 percent—a fair profit—and charges a $3 pharmacy fee and a $5 shipping fee. Take the generic estradiol cream for which Dr. Casperson's pharmacy tried to charge her a copay of $265. That same vaginal estrogen on Cuban's website costs about $25.

It's worth keeping an eye on the prescription marketplace, as options are changing—and so are prices. For example, the U.K. has been providing vaginal estrogen over the counter since September 2022, a move the British Menopause Society called a "landmark reclassification."

6ME

what MEN *are*

BY **MITCH LITTLE**

sharing about NOPAUSE

A few things they're learning now that they've woken up to, too

True story, not so long ago, I read a letter to 587,000 strangers on Instagram. It was from my perimenopausal wife, Riss, of things she wanted me to stop doing:

Your do-not list: Read this, memorize it, maybe even frame it if necessary.

Do not touch the air conditioner or mode on the fan at bedtime. I don't care if you're cold. I'm a human furnace trapped in an emotional escape room. Wear warmer PJs, hug the dog, or go sleep in the oven. Just don't touch it.

Do not say, "Are you okay?" No, I am not. I was okay ten minutes ago, then I wasn't. Then I cried. Then I laughed. Now I'm furious and possibly hangry, asking me to explain it will end in tears. Yours, mine, possibly both, I can't say.

Do not comment on the snack stash. Yes, that is my third bag of fun-size chips. Yes, I'm eating peanut butter with a soup ladle instead of a teaspoon. The snacks are sacred. Back away slowly. In fact, you can just not touch them at all.

Do not attempt to fix my mood. I'm not a broken printer. I don't need troubleshooting. Just a nod. Murmur, "You're amazing," and maybe hand me a blanket and a cookie. Preferably whilst backing out of the room.

Do not say it's probably just hormones. Let me stop you right there. That phrase is a one-way ticket to sleeping in the car with the windows up. Did I mention it's summer?

Do not use the word "cranky" to describe me. In fact, just stop doing that. Try passionately aggressive. Try deeply introspective. Try silence. Silence is good. Silence will save you.

Do not assume we're out of the woods. Some days, I'm calm. Some days a war. Treat every day like a surprise fire drill, and you'll be fine.

Do not forget I still love you. Underneath the meltdowns and wildly fluctuating moods, I'm still me, just with less estrogen and more opinions.

Love always,
Your glorious, unpredictable, occasionally weepy, hormonally hijacked wife.

Confession: When you went to Canada, you thought you were going for two weeks. I told you, "No, babe, the three-week flights are cheaper. Way more worthwhile." Yeah, that was a bold-faced lie. They were actually more expensive—like, way more expensive. Moral of the story, never underestimate how far I'll go for sacred, glorious, do-not-disturb-me alone time. I will lie to get this.

P.S. You may now bring me chocolate and step away.

Why was I reading such a letter on Instagram? Let's jump back 15 years ago, when I was a little bit lost and trying to find my feet. I didn't know what I wanted to do, right? So I got a job working as a *glassy*—that's an Australian slang term for somebody who picks up empty glasses at a bar, like a barback.

On my second day of work, at about 5 p.m. on a Saturday afternoon, in walks this woman. *She was stunning. Head-to-toe perfection.* There was a party scheduled for that night, and she was the first guest to arrive. She later told me that her ambition was to be the first one in so she could be the first one out. But as the night went on, we ended up chatting a lot. I remember asking myself, "How am I going to get this woman's number?" As it happened, she passed it to me before she left.

We've been together ever since. I'm a father to a 15-year-old boy and stepfather to my 20-year-old stepson and 26-year-old stepdaughter. Just to give you some context into our household, my wife is 11 years older than me. So that's how, as a 36-year-old, I can have a stepdaughter who's 26 and a stepson who's 20. We've been very happy—my wife has a fantastic job, the kids are doing well, the older two are now both full-time employees in my business in the health and fitness industry.

It's been an amazing life.

Except somewhere along the line, it became less amazing for my wife.

I think this is a typical bloke thing—being a little bit slower off the mark and perhaps not being extremely observant—but one day it hit me. We all were in the

Alex Charfen
founder of The Brotherhood Society

Brother, this is why so many women leave during menopause...and no, it's not because they "lost their minds" or suddenly became selfish or got corrupted by TikTok therapists... Here's the part most men don't want to hear. For decades women have been holding the emotions load of the relationship. Regulating for both people. Softening everything. Making it work. Menopause doesn't create dissatisfaction. It removes the buffer that was hiding it. So when a woman hits this phase and looks around and thinks, "I'm tired." "I'm done managing this." "I can't keep carrying both of us." What she's really saying is "I no longer have the biology to survive an uncontained relationship." Menopause is a truth serum. If the relationship is grounded, safe, regulated, it often deepens. If it's chaotic, reactive, or dependent on her emotional labor, it collapses. This isn't about blaming women. And it's not about shaming men. It's a warning. If your relationship only works because she is absorbing instability, biology will eventually collect the bill. Masculine leadership isn't about control. It's about regulation. The men who survive this chapter don't get louder. They get steadier. And that makes all the difference. Here's the part nobody wants to say out loud: Many marriages don't survive menopause because the woman finally runs out of hormones that were compensating for a man who never learned how to regulate. That's not an insult. That's biology.

Jesse Robertson
@husbands4menopause

Husbands, do you even know what menopause is—or is your wife going through hell by herself?

kitchen, and my wife laughed and smiled. And I realized that I hadn't seen her laugh or her huge smile in, well, I couldn't remember how long. She was once known for her joy—her nickname was Smiley. I started to be a little bit more observant about how she was doing, noticing that she was a bit crankier than usual, a little bit short tempered.

During those months and years, I genuinely mean this, I thought that my wife didn't like me anymore. I thought that I annoyed her. I thought that I'd done something wrong. Her unhappiness left me guessing, "What did I do? What have I done? Have I done something bad?"

Then I came home one day and didn't see her downstairs. I called out for her. No answer. I looked around the house and yard but didn't see her—that was weird. I finally went upstairs and found her sitting on the bed in tears. I cannot express how out of character this was. I asked her if she was okay, and she said she'd had a moment earlier that day where she thought that the only way out of her mind and the way that she was feeling was to take her own life.

That was something I *never* expected my wife to say.

And that was the moment I realized two things: The first is that there was something bigger going on. The second was that I knew nothing—absolutely zero—about what my wife was going through. Sure, I understood that menopause was a thing, but if you asked me about it back then, I would've said something like, "It's when women

Joe Warner
Burning Up, Frozen Out

The good news for you is that you don't need any grand gestures, you don't need to fix anything, and you don't need to have all of the answers. In fact, you don't need any of the answers. All you need to do is show up.... Ask, "Is there anything I can do today to help?" She might say no, but it might just open a line of communication that's been shut for weeks or even months.

get hot, I think?" So I started to look into what happens to women in midlife, and I learned that perimenopause and menopause isn't something that's widely spoken about. Not only do a lot of women not understand much about it, neither do doctors or GPs. This is where the problem starts. We've got educated medical professionals who are sending women from one doctor to the next. I tell everyone that I'm not an expert, but at this point, I think *I* could sit in a doctor's office and be more helpful: "Oh, well, Cheryl, you're 45. The reason you're feeling the way you're feeling is because you're going through perimenopause. You've got no sex hormones. There's no wonder you feel terrible. I'm going to send you to my specialist. We're going to get you in a better position."

It's quite frustrating, and I'll give one example of why: Not only did my wife battle poor mental health for many, many, many years, she's also experienced physical repercussions from the neglect of medical professionals. Nobody gave her the advice that she needed. They would just prescribe her things like B12 or injections that didn't have any impact on what she really needed. Let me tell you that you can take as much vitamin C or vitamin D as you want, but what a woman actually needs is somebody who understands what's happening to her body at midlife. By the time my wife finally found the right care, she had practically no estrogen, no progesterone, no testosterone. Despite having been physically active her whole life, she got diagnosed six months ago

"Here's what I've learned about perimenopause: My wife is **losing every chemical** that her body gave her to be **able to stand me.** So I'm going through a **midlife crisis** and she's going through **perimenopause,** and the only thing we have in common is we're **both thinking about me dying.**"

—DUSTIN NICKERSON,
COMEDIAN

with osteoporosis in her hip and lower back. If she'd been prescribed estrogen years ago and had the appropriate levels of estrogen and sex hormones running through her body, this would not have been the case.

As a husband, when someone you care about isn't treated well, you start to have these vigilante feelings—you want to go put on a cape and start taking down the world.

Or in my case, you start sharing what you were learning on your socials. I didn't post Reels to gain followers or an audience or even raise awareness. I was using my phone almost like a diary to get some thoughts and emotions off my chest. I did not expect in a million years for it to generate as much traction or as much attention as it did.

But I kind of understand it. After all, when do men ever get spoken to in regards to women's hormones and transitions? We don't know about our partner's menstrual cycles. We don't know about the hormonal changes they have during perimenopause or menopause. We don't know that the divorce rates or suicide rates tend to peak for women in midlife.

Understanding all this has made a huge difference for my wife and me. She will openly admit, "I know yesterday I was so short and so rude with you and so awful, but I just didn't have the energy to turn up and be bubbly and patient and nice." And for me, I'm just like, "Look, I get it. I get it. I know you don't hate me. You hate perimenopause." It's all good.

Which is not to say it's all perfect.

We still butt heads, we still have our arguments, we're still human beings, but for the most part, we've got an understanding of what's going on. I'm able to say to my wife, "You know what? I understand that you're going through this. I understand that you had a bad night's sleep, but *that* wasn't called for." She can hear that. We can even have a little bit of a joke about it.

The posts I do for social media have also given us the opportunity to have a bit of fun. It's fun to come up with some of the concepts. It's fun to shoot them. It's fun for me to ask my wife for another list of things I do that drive her insane. Did I mention the letter I read was the *fifth* one she'd written? (At my request, to be clear, though she hasn't yet said she was out of material.)

Sharing these moments on my socials (@mitchlittleacademy) means I get messages from a lot of women. Believe it or not, my wife is fine with dozens of ladies' comments on my account, because as she reads through their thoughts and experiences, she feels more connected and less alone than she once did.

I've also heard from a lot of men. They say how difficult it is to see their partners in physical and emotional pain and not understand why. Or how hard it is to see a version of their wife starting to slip away. They feel a little bit lost, a little bit alone. They send

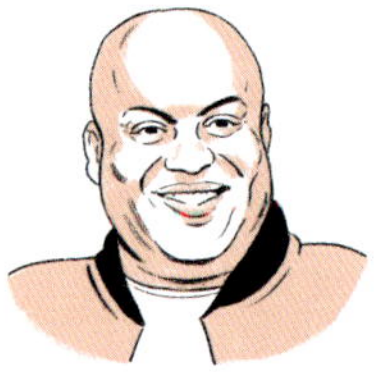

"I'm going to do a little bit more communicating as I see these symptoms coming along, because right now we've still got young kids. We're busy. It's easy for me to overlook any kind of behavioral changes because we're running around. It's easy for her to overlook it, too."

—CRAIG ROBINSON,
ON *IMO*, THE PODCAST HE HOSTS WITH HIS SISTER MICHELLE OBAMA

me messages, like, "I thought that I was the only one experiencing this." Or, "I had no idea that that is what my wife is going through." One guy commented on a Reel: "Needs to be more of this content helping us guys learn to be better without judgment." In another video, I gave advice to the fellas, including "any form of breathing, especially from the nostrils is now out of bounds." It was a lighthearted way to connect. Women dropped a ton of smiley emojis, added more suggestions, and tagged their partners. A number of men jumped on the joke too, adding some of the things they no longer do because it annoys their wives, like one guy who said, "I sleep outside in a tree house i built 30ft up and my breathing still annoys her, but I never knew blinking was so loud, 🤣🤣🤣🤣"

Listen, relationships during perimenopause and menopause can take a bit of a hit. But I do believe that if you understand what's happening, you can become closer. I feel that my job is to be my wife's bodyguard, because if not me, then who? Being the person who's not going to allow my wife to have poor mental health, to have poor muscle mass, to have poor bone density—that's a role that I take extremely seriously because I want my wife to have the best possible quality of life.

Trust me, if you can talk to your partner, it just makes everything so much better. That means checking in. That means paying a little bit closer attention. If I know that my wife has had a poor night's sleep or that she's got a headache, I'm going to make an effort to be a little bit less annoying or pick up the slack around the house—basically, not be a man baby. Because perimenopause or menopause is not a solo sport. It takes a team, so fellas, grab your partner by the hand, and support her through this time.

Michael Hunter
@upspiral.life

Menopause isn't a crisis—it's a coronation. If your partner is going through menopause, and you're wondering what happened to the woman you married, she didn't vanish. She's evolving.... What she's doing is not drama; it's biochemistry and betrayal from within her own body. Estrogen is leaving the chat; progesterone ghosted her months ago, and now her adrenal glands are expected to fill in for the entire endocrine department. And what does she get for all that? Insomnia, brain fog, rage, dryness, and sadness. What else does she get? A society that whispers, "She's just getting old." Like it's a moral failure. Let me make it really plain for you: This is not the time for you to withdraw, mock, fix, or "give her space." This is the time for you to show up. Can you handle it when she says, "I don't need your opinion"? Can you hold her when she can't hold herself? Can you resist saying, "You were never like this before"? And instead say, "I'm here for you now"? She doesn't need a critic. She needs a teammate. And guess what? She's not broken. She's transforming, because this is a furnace that creates queens. If you can stay steady through the fire, you're not just going to get her back, you're going to get her reborn. She's going to be wiser, clearer, and unapologetically done with nonsense. It's pretty refreshing.... You're not losing your woman. You're witnessing the unveiling of a masterpiece. If you play it right, it might just be the most powerful love story yet.

what if MENOPA
were your RENAISS

BY **ANNE FULENWIDER**

7

USE

SANCE?

Your Next Era

Years ago, when middle age seemed like it only happened to other people, I took an Ashtanga yoga class in Montauk, New York. As I clumsily shifted from downward dog to chaturanga, I noticed an older woman at the front of class, with gray braids, a purple T-shirt, and lithe taut limbs. She seemed to swim from pose to pose, as graceful as a seal in water. A beatific peace emanated from her that I have been thinking about more and more as I enter this next decade: 50. A friend's older sister recently told her that "after 50, you can kiss your beauty goodbye." Could that be true? I may be naive, stubborn, and vain, but I refuse to accept this pronouncement. I don't aspire to be one of those "well-preserved" faces of the Upper East Side or Beverly Hills. I want to become some version of that beautiful wise yoga sage, but how?

A few years ago, I started a morning regimen of 25 minutes of yoga and five minutes of meditation. Brief, achievable, and surprisingly helpful in many ways. I kept to it for quite a while, maybe 18 months, and even started to find a little inner peace, or at least mental clarity. But it became much harder to summon the will once I entered perimenopause. For me, the onslaught arrived in the form of anxiety, intense mood swings, alternating bouts of tears and rage, sleeplessness, and weight gain. I thought I was going crazy.

Theories abound about why we experience this transition. Women are living longer than we used to, and maybe evolution hasn't worked quickly enough for our bodies to catch up to our extended life expectancy. There is probably something to be learned from the killer whales of the Pacific, one of the only species aside from humans to experience menopause. Well past the end of their reproductive years, female orcas lead the young male whales in their pods on expeditions across the ocean, showing them the best hunting territories—sharing wisdom hard-won over long lives.

For me, the best thing about getting older is a thrilling, newfound F-it kind of confidence; the certainty that I am absolutely done worrying about what everyone else thinks. Nonetheless, I have to admit that the visible, physical effects of aging really sting. Losing hair in the shower, or glimpsing a little too much scalp at the part, can ruin a morning. And enough about the well-earned lines in our faces and the graceful aging of older French film stars. Sure, there is much to embrace about our lengthening

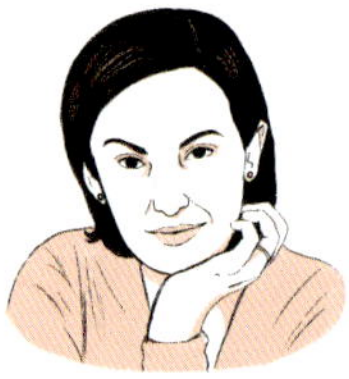

"One of the more surprising things I've learned is that postmenopausal women are generally happier than younger ones—and generally happier than they themselves were before menopause."

—LISA MOSCONI, PHD, *THE MENOPAUSE BRAIN*

lives, our accumulated wisdom, our sorting out of what's important in life. But no one likes to think of their skin as "crepey." One beautiful friend recently lamented the quality of the skin around her hips and abdomen. Another deplores her "bat wings." These body parts are not the public billboards that our faces are; these are more private sources of mourning and self-flagellation.

My best friend from childhood and I found ourselves pregnant with our first children at the same time. We traded daily phone calls to bemoan the secret horrors of pregnancy. "Hemorrhoids? Now we're getting hemorrhoids?" she began one conversation. "There's just this endless parade of indignities that no one warned us about." Our mothers, hers a stunning, blonde Eastern European and mine a sunny American, prone to glorifying, had definitely not been forthcoming with the details of this stage of life. But if the not-so-pretty surprises of childbearing were something our mothers glossed over, they buried the indignities of perimenopause and menopause deep in the ground and threw away the shovel. There's no asking them now. Mine is gone; my best friend's, fading into the fog of memory loss.

These days there are lots of people trying to help us ease this transition. There are teas, powders, gratitude journals, nutrition coaches, and wellness retreats. There are book groups, podcasts, and apps. Many of them are helpful. As we continue to extend our lifespans, we will have to figure out how to live better, healthier, and happier. Some of that is a mystery to be puzzled out collectively, in the company of others on the journey. A big part of the solution, however, is based in science that has been with us for decades.

The evidence is now clear, and the experts, including those at the American College of

Obstetricians and Gynecologists and the North American Menopause Society, agree: For the vast majority of healthy women, the benefits of menopausal hormone therapy started within 10 years of menopause far outweigh the risks. Period. And the lack of clarity on this topic has caused much harm.

When I realized the extent of the misinformation around menopause, I knew I had to do more than call my best friend and bitch about my mood swings (though I did that, too). I started a company with a friend who endured surgical menopause at 40. In our online support groups and live events, week after week, we've heard the stories of women who have suffered intensely for years, who are profoundly relieved to have found answers and solutions to their symptoms. In living rooms and auditoriums around the country, we've heard stories of relationships repaired, marriages saved (or finally abandoned), lives won back, and, over and over again, joy reclaimed. The experience has been beyond gratifying, and six years after leaving my magazine career to launch a women's health company serving women in midlife and menopause, I am now on hormone therapy and much better for it. Symptoms solved, I can fully engage in this profoundly liberating era of life.

"Aging is the extraordinary process where you become the person you always should have been." The David Bowie quote has become an anthem for the newly menopausal. It's not that the earlier versions of ourselves were false. It's just that, having spent decades twisting ourselves into every possible contortion of who others thought we should be, we've finally come to the exhilarating conclusion that the only possible path forward is to embrace our authentic selves. It's got

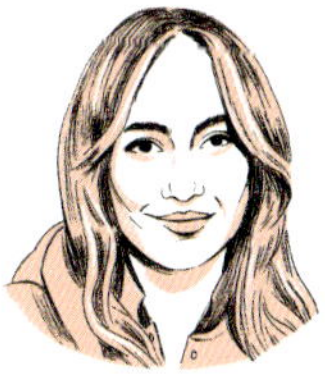

"When I turned 40, I was like, 'Huh. I accept myself more now.' It was much more comforting."

—JENNIFER LOPEZ,
ON *TODAY*

“**I love not getting my period.** There—I said it.... My first Memorial Day through Labor Day after menopause... it was the **summer of the white pant.**”

—KELLY RIPA,
ON HER PODCAST
LET’S TALK OFF CAMERA

something to do with biology, for sure. ("This must be what it feels like to be a MAN," one friend proclaimed triumphantly of her bold new confidence and freedom from menstruation.) But something else is happening, too. So many women have come to Alloy, as patient or employee, and shared something like, "What I've been doing so far no longer feels right, and I've decided to make a change" or "I want to spend my time doing something more meaningful to me." Intention over convention has emerged as a theme.

The Great Menopausal Awakening of the 2020s is good for so many things: for women finding community and not suffering in isolation, and for broadcasting the knowledge that safe, excellent solutions exist. But let's not let the pure joy awaiting everyone who gets a handle on their biology and steps unhindered into this magical time get lost in the noise.

My grandmother lived to 101, and in her mid-50s, after two husbands and seven children, she decided to travel to India and Japan to study Buddhism. At around the same age, my mother, who had left college at 19, decided to complete her degree. And in my mid-40s, I left a 25-year career in media to pursue a career in women's health. Not all midlife awakenings need show up as a dramatic change in direction. Many of us find solace in a simple shift in perspective. I've recently discovered gardening, and a new appreciation of green spaces. I go on more walks. My friends and I have started an annual hiking trip. And I've returned to the yoga and meditation apps. Have I achieved purple yoga sage–level enlightenment or the grace and laser-sharp precision of the orcas? Not quite. But do I believe I've kissed beauty goodbye? Not a chance.

The spark I glimpsed all those years ago in the yoga studio came from something that has nothing to do with taut skin or plump lips, and more to do with joy, light, flow, a comfort with sex, your body and pleasure, and a sense of finally belonging. Another magnetic older woman I remember so clearly from years ago was seated across from me on the subway one evening on my commute home. She had a silver-white bob, blue eyes, and sapphire rings, and was surrounded by family. Her face was lined, her eyes shining. As I stared at her, trying to divine the secret to her buoyant equanimity, she smiled at me, and I glimpsed the beautiful badassery of a chieftainess. She was simply magnificent. I hold her and the Montauk yoga sage as beacons from years ahead, models of who I can still be, and I can't wait.

Anne Fulenwider is the former editor in chief of Marie Claire *and the cofounder of Alloy Health, a digital health platform helping midlife women thrive.*

8

what

COMES

NEXT

Advances in perimenopause and menopause care in the near (and slightly later) future

It's an unfortunate (and infuriating) reality that despite women making up roughly half of the global population, only a small fraction of biomedical research funding goes toward female-specific conditions beyond cancer and fertility issues. One 2025 analysis suggests that less than 1 percent of pharmaceutical research dollars go to non-cancer women's health issues. As a result, so many of the health concerns that uniquely affect us remain poorly understood and hard to treat.

When it comes to menopause, the research status quo is finally starting to change, in part because it has become harder to ignore. (Kudos to Gen Xers and older Millennials who refuse to navigate this transition in silence.) None of this fixes decades of neglect overnight, but it does change what's possible. More funding means better data, better tools, and more ambitious questions—not just about symptoms, but about long-term health trajectories. Here's what some experts predict will change about how women will experience the menopause transition.

Harnessing AI to Predict Perimenopause

One of the most frustrating parts of perimenopause is that a woman won't know when it will start, how long it will last, or what specific symptoms she will experience until she's in it. Even then, it can be confusing: Is it The Change, or is it stress, illness, infection, an autoimmune disorder, thyroid issues...or even a surprise pregnancy?! But experts hope soon to harness the power of technology to predict when perimenopause will strike. Last year, neuroscientist Frida Polli, PhD, launched Female Medicine Through Machine Learning (FMML), a research program that aims to leverage artificial intelligence to rapidly comb through massive data sets of real-world biological data—50 percent of which come from women. One use of this tech is to look for patterns that show unexpected signifiers of perimenopause, says David Pépin, PhD, the head of ovarian research at FMML. Since AI makes it easier and faster to analyze large sets of data, "you can just look at everything—not just hormones or other signs of aging, but all kinds of health indicators you wouldn't necessarily think of," says Pépin, who is also an associate professor of surgery at Harvard Medical School and the associate director of the Pediatric Surgical Research Laboratories at Massachusetts General Hospital.

A hypothetical example: We know that the menopause transition is a time when a woman's cardiovascular risk increases, Polli says; retinal scanning is showing some promise in predicting that kind of risk. In the future, we could incorporate information from a routine retinal scan, along with a myriad of other factors (say, blood cholesterol data) to help a woman understand how menopause is affecting her and what symptoms to expect. Her doctor could use that information to help guide interventions and treatment. "This is the power of machine learning: aggregating disparate data into clinically actionable predictions that, in conjunction with doctors' oversight, will revolutionize treatment," says Polli.

"The therapeutic part is farther in the future," Pépin adds, "but many clinics are already starting to experiment with AI." He predicts that more health care centers will start using algorithms for this purpose within the next two years.

A Hot Flash Treatment That Sounds Like Science Fiction

It seems almost insulting to ask a woman engulfed in a hot flash to imagine she's standing in the cold. But what if she could step into an immersive experience designed not just to cool the senses, but to teach the brain how to respond differently to hot flashes when they strike? That's the idea behind a program in development by women's health researchers from the Mayo Clinic in Jacksonville, Florida, and VR experts at Cedars-Sinai in Los Angeles. Their program incorporates cognitive behavioral therapy (CBT) into an immersive experience using a virtual reality headset that offers 360-degree views of a snowy landscape and the sound of the winter wind. Through eight weeks of at-home VR experiences, users learn how to regulate stress responses and bodily sensations associated with hot flashes so it doesn't feel like a five-alarm fire when one happens.

"The goal is not simply distraction, but helping the brain reinterpret internal signals so hot flashes feel less intense and disruptive," says Stephanie Faubion, MD, the director of the Mayo Clinic's Center for Women's Health, medical director for the Menopause Society, and one of the project leaders. There is strong scientific evidence that CBT is an effective way to deal with hot flashes and night sweats; VR has already shown promise in delivering self-administered CBT for acute and chronic pain, sleep, and mood disorders. The research team will soon conduct a pilot study, says Dr. Faubion; after safety and preliminary efficacy have been established, it will do a randomized controlled trial. The researchers will also test to see if this type of program works with other perimenopause symptoms, including compromised mood, sleep, and sexual function. No hormones, no drugs—just a novel way to help the mind and body work together during menopause.

“How wonderful would it be if we could get to a place where we are able to have these **conversations openly** and **without shame**? Admit, freely, that this is what’s going on. So we don’t feel like we’re going **mad** or **insane** or **alone** in any of the symptoms we are having”

—GILLIAN ANDERSON,
TO LENNY LETTER

Sleep Relief—at Long Last!

Experts have recently realized that menopausal sleep disruptions aren't entirely due to hot flashes. Research shows that while hot flashes can disrupt women's sleep, most of their overnight awake time is due to factors other than flashes, says Pauline Maki, PhD, the director of Women's Mental Health Research Program at the University of Illinois Chicago College of Medicine. She and her fellow researchers dug into the data on the hot flash drug elinzanetant, which works on two receptors in the brain. They found that its ability to improve sleep wasn't just because it curbed hot flashes: The drug also seemed to act on additional neuroendocrine pathways linked to sleep regulation. This is promising news for the many perimenopausal women who aren't necessarily waking up with soaked-through pajamas but are continuously waking up. While elinzanetant was FDA-approved for moderate to severe menopausal hot flashes in 2025 under the name Lynkuet, new studies are underway to determine whether the drug might also enhance sleep in women who have minimal hot flashes but still have trouble getting quality shut-eye. "We're excited about the possibility that it would work in this group, but we just need a little more research," Maki says.

Tracking Changes in a Woman's Brain

To date, there have been few large, long-term studies that track changes in the female brain as a woman transitions from peri- to postmenopause. But we're finally getting some answers, says Maki. About eight years ago, researchers started collecting data from the Human Connectome Project, a massive, groundbreaking neuroimaging study, and its ongoing extension, the Aging Adult Brain Connectome project. One study using that data specifically focuses on the brain during menopause; it is following 220 women ages 40 to 59 for up to 10 years. Researchers will measure participants' brain health across the menopause transition using memory and thinking tests as well as brain imaging scans (e.g., MRI). They hope to link these changes to menopause symptoms and hormonal changes and assess risk factors for Alzheimer's over time. They'll have more than 150 data points per stage of menopause, which is unprecedentedly comprehensive. "We're just beginning to get the data to show over time what changes in the same woman as she transitions through menopause," says Maki, who is a principal investigator on the project with Susan Bookheimer, PhD, at UCLA's David Geffen School of Medicine. Over the next year or two, Maki expects to start seeing insights from the data. The ultimate goal: a new understanding of how menopause contributes to sex differences in cognitive aging and Alzheimer's disease and to identify possible targets for prevention.

Hormone Therapy to Possibly *Prevent* Breast Cancer

The infamous Women's Health Initiative study from 2002, which broadly linked hormone replacement therapy (HRT) to breast cancer, had a chilling effect on the treatment's use. (Later studies concluded that these findings were misleading.) Research has since added more nuance to the picture, showing that the type and dose of HRT, how long it is used, the women's age at which therapy begins, and breast cancer history play a role in cancer risk. What's more, a major 2024 study published in *Breast Cancer Research and Treatment* analyzed 10 randomized clinical trials and concluded that using estrogen alone, without progestin, significantly reduces breast cancer incidence. (Note: Only people who have had their uterus removed can take estrogen-only HRT.) "There is some evidence that estrogen can cause the death of breast cancer cells, which would contribute to a lower risk of breast cancer," says JoAnn Manson, MD, the chief of the division of preventive medicine at Brigham and Women's Hospital and one of the study authors. Meanwhile, a growing body of research suggests that progestins, a synthetic form of progesterone used in birth control pills and some preparations of HRT, come with an increased risk of breast cancer—and might be the reason why HRT got a bad rap. (Add to that the relatively advanced ages of the original WHI sample set.)

Dr. Manson and her team will continue to analyze the data to pinpoint risk (searching for answers to such questions as: How long is it safe to take estrogen alone? What health characteristics matter?). They're also hoping to do a new randomized trial to see how the types of HRT more commonly prescribed today (e.g., transdermal estradiol skin patches, micronized progesterone) may affect risks of breast cancer and cardiovascular disease. But that will take many years—and research dollars—to see results.

New Sources of Funding for Women's Health Research

While older health initiatives designed to better understand women's health netted hundreds of millions of federal funding in the past, new support of that magnitude is more difficult to access. Thankfully, there is still money going toward furthering menopause research. In 2024, the federal ARPA-H Sprint for Women's Health committed more than $100 million to projects tackling everything from ovarian aging to brain health and pain measurement. Private philanthropy is getting into the act, too. In 2025, Melinda French Gates's investment group Pivotal partnered with health engine nonprofit Wellcome Leap on a $100 million initiative to accelerate research in neglected areas like menopause, cardiovascular disease, and mental health. Other donors gave $20 million to the NewYork-Presbyterian hospital system to seed an integrated perimenopause-to-menopause program, and $5 million to the Menopause Society for digital education and training for healthcare professionals.

Researchers are also getting creative in how they structure their projects to get the answers we need to move women's health forward. "The landscape is changing in terms of how we do research today versus how we did it 20 or 30 years ago," says Dr. Faubion. "We are now moving to different ways to accomplish clinical trials, including more decentralized studies that we can run essentially online, and using big data sets and machine learning to answer questions that in the past would have required clinical trials to answer."

A Tool to Forecast a Woman's Health Risks

A groundbreaking study published in *BMJ Open* in 2023 developed a scoring system that can forecast midlife women's future health risks up to a decade in advance—and it may soon come to a doctor's office near you. The Study of Women's Health Across the Nation (SWAN) Seven Score is the first of its kind to predict the risk of health issues for women in the 55 to 65 age group. The tool addresses women-specific risks in the areas of educational attainment, smoking, body mass index, cardiovascular disease history, osteoarthritis, depressive systems, and overall health. In theory, a woman in menopause and her doctor could use this tool to see what her future health risks are and come up with an action plan ASAP.

Considering that many health care practitioners aren't trained in midlife women's health, this tool could make a big difference in helping women get the preventive care they didn't know they needed. Nanette Santoro, MD, an ob-gyn, professor in the division of reproductive sciences at the University of Colorado Anschutz, and chair of the translation and dissemination committee for the SWAN project, says it's high on her list to get this tool out in public, and for it to become a standard part of a midlife woman's annual checkup. That will require additional funding, which she hopes to secure soon. "Being aware of areas where there is room for improvement and managing these conditions when a woman is in her 50s is likely to pay off in terms of their future health," Dr. Santoro says.

I wouldn't get in the DeLorean and go back for anything. I've **never been happier**. I've never been **wiser**."

—DREW BARRYMORE,
TO OPRAH DAILY

A Drug to Delay Menopause… Forever?

Ten years ago, when molecular biologist Piraye Yurttas Beim, PhD, had the wildly radical idea that menopause wasn't a biological necessity and that ovarian function could be extended, people thought she was "totally crazy." Today, her biotech company Celmatix Therapeutics, which focuses on ovarian health, has made strides toward making that idea a reality—supported in part by millions of dollars in U.S. government funding (awarded in 2024). Beim's aha moment came while studying the molecular pathways that are disrupted in ovarian health conditions such as endometriosis, polycystic ovary syndrome, and menopause—pathways that are also affected by diseases like diabetes, heart disease, and autoimmune disorders. She realized that the ovaries aren't just reproductive organs but a central command center for many other aspects of women's health. For example, she notes, women who undergo early menopause have a 300 percent increased risk of multiple chronic conditions by the age of 70, including dementia, diabetes, osteoporosis, metabolic issues, and autoimmune conditions. As such, Beim believes that women should have gonads (i.e., ovaries) that function throughout life, just like men's. Currently, Beim is working on a drug that targets anti-Müllerian hormone, a protein produced in your ovaries that controls the growth of egg follicles for ovulation. The drug would slow the release of eggs from the ovaries, putting the brakes on ovarian aging. The idea, Beim says, is that a woman would start taking this drug early in life, come off it when she wanted to have a baby, then go back on it to have a "smooth glide" into aging, without the hormonal havoc of perimenopause. If the treatment pans out, full menopause could be delayed for decades—or even become optional.

Beim says the team is weeks ahead of schedule on technical development, and their next phase is to test the drug in animals to ensure that it's safe and working as expected. (Human trials won't begin for another few years.) "I think that regulating the ovarian follicle is going to be as fundamental of a breakthrough for women's health as the birth control pill was last century," she says.

Continuing the Conversation

BY OPRAH WINFREY

Over the past few years, it's been really heartening for me to see how many women have come up to me to say that they're going through the big M, because it's a subject that I have to say has been shrouded in silence for far too long. As I've shared, when I went through it, I had major heart palpitations, couldn't concentrate, and other symptoms, but one of the tougher parts was being one of the only people speaking out about it—there was still such secrecy about it.

I'm glad to see the tide is turning. To everybody out there in the throes of this thing—the change—I say, welcome. Welcome to the club, ladies. Please know you don't have to suffer in silence. There is real help available right now. You have options—medical, holistic, emotional—and you deserve care that honors your whole self.

I also want to say this: Stay informed. Because things are changing. Doctors are being educated on this phase of life (slowly). Science is starting to catch up to what women have been saying for decades. Even legislation is starting to reflect the understanding that menopause is not a footnote—it's a major life transition that deserves support, research, and respect. What we know today is already different from what we knew five years ago, and more is coming.

I want to thank all the experts who've made it their mission to educate us all about this phase of life and contributed their wisdom to Oprah Daily and O, *the Oprah Magazine*. I also want to applaud anybody who speaks about what they're going through because the more people who share their experiences, the more we can shake off the stigma that so many women still face. Every conversation you have, every question you ask, every time you speak your truth—it all adds to a growing momentum. And my hope is that because of that momentum, the next generation of women won't be confused or blindsided or left wondering what's happening to their bodies. They'll be informed. They'll be prepared. And they'll know they're not alone.

Further Reading

Insightful books to help you understand, navigate, and thrive through midlife

The Hormone Shift
by Tasneem Bhatia, MD

A practical guide to restoring hormonal balance to improve energy, mood, metabolism, and long-term health during midlife by an integrative medicine physician specializing in endocrine balance and chronic disease prevention.

Hagitude
by Sharon Blackie

A psychologist and mythologist explores midlife as a powerful, transformative stage for women, reframing aging through myth, story, and purpose.

Estrogen Matters
by Avrum Bluming, MD, and Carol Tavris, PhD

A pioneering, science-based reassessment of estrogen therapy by an oncologist who was among the first to challenge the misinterpretation of the WHI study, explaining estrogen's critical role in women's long-term health, longevity, and disease prevention.

The Menopause Moment
by Kelly Casperson, MD

A candid guide to navigating menopause with confidence, clarity, and evidence-based care by a urologist specializing in female sexual health.

All In Her Head
by Elizabeth Comen, MD
An examination of medical bias against women by a breast oncologist and medical historian.

How to Menopause
by Tamsen Fadal
A practical, she's-been-there menopause guide by a journalist and patient advocate focused on awareness and self-advocacy.

The Menopause Manifesto
by Jen Gunter, MD
A myth-busting menopause guide by a board-certified OB-GYN known for pushing back on misinformation about menopause and empowering women with medical facts.

The New Menopause and
The New Perimenopause
by Mary Claire Haver, MD
Examinations of the menopause and perimenopause transitions, each focused on symptom relief, metabolic health, and healthy aging by an OB-GYN.

Grown Women Talk
by Sharon Malone, MD
A straight-talking menopause guide by a board-certified OB-GYN and longtime women's health advocate.

The Menopause Brain
by Lisa Mosconi, PhD
A researched-based exploration of menopause by a neuroscientist specializing in women's brain health and Alzheimer's prevention.

The Wisdom of Menopause
by Christiane Northrup, MD
An early, influential menopause perspective by one of the first OB-GYNs to popularize menopause in mainstream culture, integrating mind-body-spirit approaches to women's health.

Age Like a Girl
by Dr. Mindy Pelz

A fasting and nutrition-based longevity guide by a chiropractor focused on female health, proposing lifestyle changes aimed at supporting metabolic flexibility and brain function during this transition.

Hormone Havoc
by Amy Shah, MD

A symptom-solving hormone protocol by a dual-trained internist and nutrition specialist.

Generation M
by Jessica Shepherd, MD

A modern menopause reframing by an OB-GYN specializing in preventive care and women's longevity.

Millennial Menopause
by Lauren A. Tetenbaum, LCSW, JD, PMH-C

A mental-health-first menopause guide by a licensed therapist specializing in reproductive mood disorders.

Dare I Say It
by Naomi Watts

A stigma-breaking menopause memoir by an actress and public advocate.

Unbreakable
by Vonda Wright, MD

A strength and longevity guide by an orthopedic surgeon specializing in women's musculoskeletal aging.

Acknowledgments

Thank you to our contributors at Oprah Daily and the experts who have helped us build a national conversation on perimenopause and menopause.

Lisa Arbetter
Jennifer Ashton, MD
Naomi Barr
Leslie Baumann, MD
Esther Blum, MS, RD, CDN, CNS
Roberta Diaz Brinton, PhD
Liz Brody
Isabel Burton
Kaitlin Casaletto, PhD
Kelly Casperson, MD
Elizabeth Comen, MD
Joseph Conger, DPT
Deborah Copaken
Daniel Croley, DMD
Doris Day, MD
Sarah De La Torre, MD
Krista Bennett Demaio
Kristi Tough DeSapri, MD
Gary Elkins, PhD
Tania Elliott, MD
Dendy Engelman, MD
Tamsen Fadal
Stephanie Faubion, MD
Shelley Flannery
Eleni N. Gage
Suzanne Gilberg-Lenz, MD
Leslie Goldman
Jill Goldstein, MD
Mary Claire Haver, MD
Jill Herzig
Heather Hirsch, MD
Rosie Hopegood
Alisa Hrustic
Cassie Hurwitz
Tara K. Iyer, MD, MSCP
Beth Janes
Somi Javaid, MD
Judith Joseph, MD

Jewel Kling, MD, MPH
Audrey Kunin, MD
Pooja Lakshmin, MD
Hallie Levine
Suzanne Levine, DPM
Debra Lin, PhD
Sofia Lodato
Pauline Maki, PhD
Sharon Malone, MD
JoAnn Manson, MD
Christina Manian, RDN
Vivian Manning-Schaffel
Ellen Marmur, MD
Melissa Melby, PhD
Erin Michos, MD
Mary Jane Minkin, MD
Lisa Mosconi, PhD
Lisa Mulcahy
Jessica Nazzaro, DO
Akiko Okifuji, PhD
Mindy Pelz, DC
David Pépin, PhD
Corrie Pikul
JoAnn Pinkerton, MD
Frida Polli, PhD
Elizabeth Poynor, MD
Meghan Rabbitt
Harita Raja, MD
Amanda Robb
Rachel Rubin, MD
Nanette Santoro, MD
Jessica Shepherd, MD
Natalie H. Strand, MD
Lauren Streicher, MD
Wendy Suzuki, PhD
Lauren A. Tetenbaum, LCSW
Rebecca C. Thurston, PhD
Jessica Tomazic, MD
Fiorella Valdesolo
Jessie Van Amburg
Rhonda Voskuhl, MD
Miriam T. Weber, PhD
Jennifer Weiss-Wolf
Angela Weyand, MD
Makeba Williams, MD
Vonda Wright, MD
Piraye Yurttas Beim, PhD

Index

C

D

E

F

G

H

I

J

K

L

M

R

S

HEARST HOME

This book is intended as a reference volume only, not as a medical manual. The information given here is designed to help you make informed decisions about your health. It is not intended as a substitute for any treatment that may have been prescribed by your doctor. If you suspect that you have a medical problem, we urge you to seek competent medical help.

Library of Congress Cataloging-in-Publication Data
Available on Request

10 9 8 7 6 5 4 3 2 1

Published by Hearst Home, an imprint of
Hearst Books/Hearst Magazine Media, Inc.
300 W 57th Street
New York, NY 10019

For information about custom editions, special sales, premium and corporate purchases:
hearst.com/magazines/hearst-books

Printed in China
978-1-958395-47-9

CREDITS

Illustrations by Jessica Bromer
Cover concept by Shubhani Sarker